AUDIOLOGY
THE FUNDAMENTALS

AUDIOLOGY
THE FUNDAMENTALS

Fred H. Bess, Ph.D.

Division of Hearing and Speech Sciences
Vanderbilt University School of Medicine
and
Bill Wilkerson Hearing and Speech Center
Nashville, Tennessee

Larry E. Humes, Ph.D.

Department of Speech and Hearing Sciences
Indiana University
Bloomington, Indiana

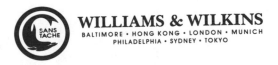

WILLIAMS & WILKINS
BALTIMORE · HONG KONG · LONDON · MUNICH
PHILADELPHIA · SYDNEY · TOKYO

Editor: John P. Butler
Associate Editor: Linda Napora
Project Editor: Miriam L. Kleiger
Designer: Jo Anne Janowiak
Illustration Planner: Ray Lowman
Production Coordinator: Charles E. Zeller

Copyright © 1990
Williams & Wilkins
428 East Preston Street
Baltimore, Maryland 21202, USA

Accurate indications, adverse reactions, and dosage schedules for drugs are provided in this book, but it is possible that they may change. The reader is urged to review the package information data of the manufacturers of the medications mentioned.

Printed in the United States of America
Library of Congress Cataloging in Publication Data
Bess, Fred H.
   Audiology : the fundamentals / Fred H. Bess, Larry E. Humes.
      p.   cm.
   Bibliography: p.
   Includes index.
   ISBN 0-683-00619-3
   1. Audiology.   I. Humes, Larry.   II. Title.
   [DNLM: 1.   Audiology.   WV 270 B557a]
RF290.B44 1990
617.8—dc20
DNLM/DLC
for Library of Congress   89-5752
                                                                                  CIP

                                                                              92   93
                                              3   4   5   6   7   8   9   10

To our wives, Susie and Marty;
our parents; and
our children—
Danny, Amy, Andy, and Lauren

PREFACE

Audiology: The Fundamentals offers a contemporary treatment of the profession of audiology at the introductory level. Indeed, we found writing this book to be a difficult task. Although audiology is a relative newcomer to the health care professions, it is a dynamic discipline that has undergone rapid change and growth since its inception during World War II. Because of these transformations, as well as space limitations, we found ourselves forced to make choices regarding which areas of audiology to include in an undergraduate text. We have chosen to discuss those topics that are most important to the beginning student rather than to provide a cursory review of the broad scope of the profession.

This book was written for three reasons. First, we believe there is a need for an introductory book that provides a contemporary approach to audiology: one that strikes a balance between the traditional concepts and newer developments in the profession. Second, we believe there is a place for an introductory book that considers the type of student typically enrolled in a beginning audiology course. Our experience suggests that most students taking an introductory course in audiology are planning careers in either speech-language pathology or special education. With this in mind, we have tried to emphasize material on auditory pathology in children, especially middle ear disease, and we have included chapters on screening auditory function and education for the hearing impaired. Hopefully, such information will be of value to students when they begin practicing their chosen profession. We have also attempted to present the material in an easy-to-read, easy-to-understand style. References are intentionally omitted from the body of the book with the exception of direct quotations. Vignettes are used generously throughout the text to enhance interest, to provide illustrative examples of ideas, and to crystallize definitions of difficult-to-grasp concepts. Finally, we wanted to share with the beginning student our enthusiasm for audiology and, more importantly, the challenges and rewards associated with this health-related discipline. We sincerely hope that this book will enhance enthusiasm and motivate students to pursue a career in audiology.

The book is divided into three sections. The first section provides background information on the profession of audiology and a basic review of the underlying principles of acoustics and the anatomy and physiology of the auditory system. A general understanding of Section 1 is essential to the practice of the profession of audiology. Section 2 is concerned with the principles of audiologic measurement and the general application of audiologic procedures. Toward this end, Section 2 focuses on basic measurement of auditory function, auditory pathologies and their associated audiologic manifestations, and screening for hearing loss and middle ear disease. Section 3 is directed at providing a general understanding of rehabilitative approaches used with hearing-impaired children and adults and the status of education for the hearing impaired.

The preparation of this book was an arduous endeavor and could not have been completed without the generous help and support of many individuals. Kathy Hollis expertly and cheerfully prepared on a timely basis numerous working drafts, as well as the final version of the book. Don Riggs developed most of the graphs and charts used throughout the book, and Doris Wasserman prepared many of the anatomic drawings. Several individuals reviewed the book or portions of the book and offered insightful analysis and suggestions for improvement. They include: Gene W. Bratt, Thomas Klee, Michael J. Lichtenstein, Freeman E. McConnell, Jay W. Sanders, and four anonymous reviewers whose constructive comments strongly influenced the content of this book. John Butler, our editor, provided support and encouragement throughout the book-writing process. The staff and the faculty of the Bill Wilkerson Hearing and Speech Center, Vanderbilt University School of Medicine (Division of Hearing and Speech Sciences) and Indiana University (Department of Speech and Hearing Sciences) offered continued support and facilities. To all of these individuals we offer our sincere appreciation.

Finally, we take this opportunity to express our love and gratitude to our parents, Helen and Samuel H. Bess and Mary and Charles E. Humes, for their confidence, direction, and continual support.

F.H.B.
L.E.H.

CONTENTS

PART ONE
INTRODUCTION

PART TWO
ASSESSMENT OF AUDITORY FUNCTION

PART THREE
MANAGEMENT STRATEGIES

PART ONE

INTRODUCTION

CHAPTER ONE

Audiology as a Profession

The purpose of this opening chapter is to offer a general discussion and review of the profession of audiology. The discussion focuses on several areas. First, statistics on the total number of cases of hearing loss, or the prevalence of hearing loss, are reviewed. The impact of hearing loss on the well-being of the individual is also briefly described. These two areas are reviewed to give the reader some sense of the magnitude of the problem, both on a national scale and as it is experienced by the affected individuals themselves. Next, the definition and historical evolution of audiology are reviewed. Various employment opportunities in this health-related discipline are surveyed. The chapter concludes with a summary of a typical graduate training program in audiology and a description of some of the professional affiliations that audiologists find worthwhile.

OBJECTIVES

Following completion of this chapter, the reader should be able to:

- Discuss the prevalence of hearing loss and the complications associated with hearing impairment.
- Define the profession of audiology.
- Appreciate the lineage of the profession of audiology.
- Describe the employment opportunities available to the audiologist.
- Understand the academic and clinical requirements needed to become an audiologist.
- Appreciate the essential accreditations and professional affiliations important to clinical audiology.

PREVALENCE AND IMPACT OF HEARING IMPAIRMENT

Before discussing audiology as a profession, it is helpful to develop some understanding of the nature of hearing loss in the United States. The estimated prevalence, or total number of existing cases, of hearing loss varies depending on several factors. These factors include: (*a*) how hearing loss was determined (i.e., questionnaire vs. hearing test); (*b*) the criterion or formula used to define the presence of a

3

hearing impairment (severe hearing loss vs. mild); and (c) the age of the individuals within the population sampled (adults vs. children). Regardless of the methods used to determine prevalence, hearing loss is known to affect a very large segment of the population in the United States. Estimates of the prevalence and prevalence rates of hearing loss for the population as a whole, and for different age groups, are summarized in Table 1.1.

It may be noted that the total number of hearing-impaired persons in the United States is slightly more than 21 million. It also can be seen that there are some 1,203,000 young people under the age of 18 years with hearing losses reported in either one or both ears. Other studies focusing on the population under 18 years of age have estimated that there are about 56,000 children under the age of 6 years with significant hearing impairment in both ears. This means that these children exhibit a hearing deficit in both ears, with the better ear exhibiting some difficulty in hearing and understanding speech. It has also been estimated that one of every 1,000–2,000 infants is born with a severe to profound hearing loss. If young children with the milder forms of hearing loss are included, the prevalence rate is thought to involve 20–30 times more children.

Returning to the statistics shown in Table 1.1, notice that the prevalence rate for hearing loss increases with increasing age. For example, in the 19- to 44-year-old category, the prevalence rate is 49.8 per thousand; whereas for the age groups 65–74 years and 75 years or older, the prevalence rates are 261.9 per thousand and 346.9 per thousand, respectively. These statistics confirm what many of us with living grandparents and great-grandparents already know: hearing loss is commonly associated with old age. This is particularly important when one considers the current number of elderly persons in the United States and the projected growth rates of the aged population. The number of individuals over the age of 65 presently exceeds 23 million, and that figure is expected to increase to more than 50 million by the year 2025.

The preceding paragraphs have established that there are a large number of

Table 1.1
Prevalence and Prevalence Rates, According to Age for Hearing Loss in the United States[a,b]

Age Group	Prevalence	Prevalence Rate (per thousand)
All ages	21,198,000	90.7
0–18 years	1,203,000	19.2
19–44 years	4,955,000	49.8
45–64 years	7,077,000	159.0
65–74 years	4,372,000	261.9
75+ years	3,591,000	346.9

[a]Adapted from Moss AJ, Parsons VL: Current estimates from the National Health Institute Survey, United States, 1985. *Vital and Health Statistics*. Series 10, no. 160. DHHS pub no. (PHS) 86-1588. Washington, DC, Public Health Services, 1986.
[b]Data were obtained from household interviews and reflect the prevalence of hearing loss in either one or both ears.

Americans of all ages with significant hearing problems. Although statistics such as these are important, they provide little insight into the devastating impact that a significant hearing impairment can have on the individual. Children who are born with a severe or profound hearing impairment experience the greatest hardship and, under most circumstances, exhibit a significant lag in educational progress. This is because the hearing impairment interferes with the child's ability to develop language and communication skills. If the development of our language system is heavily dependent on auditory input, and auditory input is reduced or eliminated, the ability to learn language will then be drastically curtailed. To illustrate, it has been noted that the average high-school graduate from a state school for the deaf has the equivalent of an eighth-grade education. Approximately 80% of our deaf adults work in manual jobs, as compared to only one-half of the hearing population. Even the milder forms of hearing loss which may be present at birth or acquired later in life can interfere with a child's educational progress.

Children are not the only ones affected negatively by the presence of a significant hearing loss. Hearing loss in the adult can produce a number of psychosocial complications. For the elderly adult, the deterioration in hearing sensitivity and the associated problems with understanding speech are known to impact on the quality of the individual's daily living activity. That is, the elderly who are hearing impaired are more likely to have poor general health, reduced mobility, fewer excursions outside the home, fewer interpersonal contacts, more depression and anxiety, and increased tension.

In summary, hearing loss occurs in large numbers of people and affects both children and adults. In addition, the prevalence rate of hearing loss increases markedly for the elderly population. Finally, the overall impact of hearing loss is significant, causing retardation in the educational progress of children and producing serious psychosocial consequences for those who acquire hearing loss later in life.

AUDIOLOGY DEFINED

Audiology is a new health-care profession concerned with the study of both normal and disordered hearing. It evolved as a spin-off from such closely related fields as speech-language pathology, medicine, special education, psychology, and hearing aid instrumentation. In the most literal sense, the term *audiology* refers to the science of hearing. A much broader definition of audiology is: the discipline involved in the prevention, identification, and evaluation of hearing and hearing disorders, the selection and evaluation of hearing aids, and the habilitation/rehabilitation of individuals with hearing impairment. Although these definitions represent commonly accepted descriptions of the profession, they in no way reflect adequately the breadth of the field or the challenges, rewards, and self-fulfillment that can result from a career in audiology. Whether your interest centers on serving people or producing new knowledge through inquiry and study, a career in audiology has much to offer.

The profession is typically subdivided into different specialties according to the nature of the population served or the setting in which the audiologist is employed. For example, a common area of specialization is pediatric audiology, in which the focus is placed on the identification, assessment, and management of the hearing-impaired neonate, infant, and school-age child. The pediatric audiologist develops special knowledge in such areas as the causes of childhood deafness, the development of audition in children, child development, the audiologic screening and evaluation of children of different age groups, and parent counseling.

Another common specialty area is referred to as medical audiology. The medical audiologist is typically employed in a medical center and assists the physician in establishing an accurate diagnosis of an auditory disorder. Toward this end, the audiologist employs highly sophisticated and specialized tests to help pinpoint the location and cause of the hearing problem. The medical audiologist spends much of his or her time determining whether hearing loss is due to a problem in the middle ear, the inner ear, or the higher centers of the auditory system within the brainstem and cortex.

Rehabilitative audiology represents a third area of specialization that is gaining widespread popularity and acceptance. The rehabilitative audiologist is concerned with the appropriate management of an individual with a hearing deficit. It is common for the rehabilitative audiologist to specialize even further by limiting the service population to either adults or children. The rehabilitative audiologist is interested in fitting the individual with appropriate amplification, such as a personal hearing aid, to help compensate for the hearing loss. This specialist also provides the individual with information on the use and care of the hearing aid. Other services offered might include speechreading, speech remediation, auditory training, and individual and family counseling. If the audiologist specializes in the rehabilitation of children, his or her activities might also include conducting special parent-infant training programs, teaching speech and language, counseling parents, and readying the child for school.

Finally, there are some audiologists whose entire practice is in an industrial setting. These audiologists are referred to as industrial audiologists. Noise is a common by-product of our highly industrialized society. As we'll learn later, high levels of noise can produce permanent loss of hearing. Because many industries have work areas that produce high noise levels, audiologists are needed to develop programs that will protect employees from noise. Audiologists organize hearing conservation programs. These programs are designed to protect the worker from hearing loss by reducing the noise levels produced by noisy equipment, monitoring the hearing of employees, offering education on noise and its damaging effects to employees, and providing ear protection to those workers placed in high-noise areas.

HISTORICAL DEVELOPMENT OF AUDIOLOGY

Although instruments (audiometers) used to measure hearing date back to the late 1800s, the discipline of audiology essentially evolved during World War II. During and following this war, many military personnel returned from combat with significant hearing impairment resulting from exposure to the many and varied types of warfare noises. Interestingly, it was a prominent speech pathologist, Robert West, who called for his profession to expand their discipline to include the area of audition. West stated: "Many workers in the field of speech correction do not realize that the time has come for those interested in this field to expand the subject so as to include . . . problems of those defective in the perception of speech. Our job should include . . . aiding the individual to hear what he ought to hear." (From West R: The mechanical ear. *Volta Review* 35:345–346, 1936.) Although a term had not yet been coined for this new field proposed by West, there was evidence that activity and interest in hearing disorders was present as early as 1936.

There has been considerable debate over who was responsible for coining the term *audiology*. Most sources credit Norton Canfield, an otolaryngologist (ear, nose, and throat physician) and Raymond Carhart, a speech-language pathologist, for deriving the term independently of one another in 1945. Both of these men were intimately involved in planning and implementing programs in specialized aural rehabilitation hospitals established for military personnel during World War II. Today, Carhart is recognized by many as the Father of Audiology (Vignette 1.1).

PROFESSIONAL OPPORTUNITIES

As shown in Figure 1.1, the modern-day audiologist has the opportunity to work within a wide variety of employment settings. The largest number of audiologists are shown to be employed in hospitals and physicians' offices followed by university or college-based clinics and by schools. A growing number of audiologists are finding employment in military-based programs (not shown in the figure). Perhaps the most rapid increase, however, is seen in private practice. The following discussion is a more detailed presentation of the professional opportunities in audiology.

Community Hospitals and Health-Care Facilities

It is estimated that about 6% of the hospitals in the United States employ between one and four audiologists. There currently exists a steady increase in the demand for audiologic services in hospitals, long-term care facilities, and home health agencies. The increased demand for audiologists in this type of setting, especially during the past several years, may be attributed to several factors. First, there is a growing trend for hospitals to develop or enhance their rehabilitation programs because the government's reimbursement systems (e.g.,

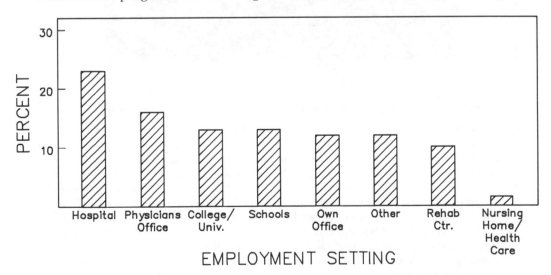

Figure 1.1.   Bar graph illustrating the distribution of employment settings for audiologists. (Adapted from Cherow E: The practice of audiology—a national perspective. *ASHA* 28:31–38, 1986.)

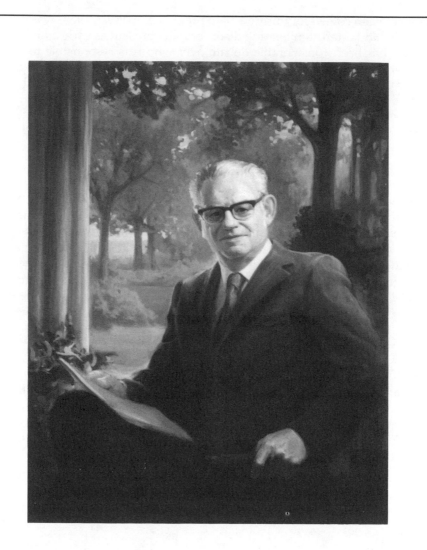

Vignette 1.1.   Raymond Carhart (1912–1975), Father of Audiology

The contributions of Dr. Raymond Carhart to the development of audiology from its earliest origins were so numerous and so significant that many think of him today as the Father of Audiology. A young professor in the School of Speech at Northwestern University when World War II broke out, he was commissioned a captain in the Army to head the Deshon General Hospital aural rehabilitation program for war-deafened military personnel at Butler, Pennsylvania. Deshon was named as one of three Army general hospitals to receive, treat, and rehabilitate soldiers who incurred hearing loss as a result of their military service. These three Army hospitals, together with the Phildelphia Naval Hospital, admitted and provided services to some 16,000 hearing-impaired enlisted and officer personnel during the course of the war.

This wartime mobilization effort served as the basis for the development of the new discipline that is now audiology. It was in 1945 that Carhart and otologist Norton Canfield are credited with coining the word *audiology* to designate the science of hearing. From the outset, Carhart recognized that the strong interprofessional relationships existing between audiology and otology must be maintained. The military program was modeled on this concept, which determined its direction for the future. As a leader in the American Speech Correction Association, Carhart was instrumental in changing the name to the American Speech and Hearing Association soon after the close of World War II. He was, moreover, one of the association's most effective liaison agents between audiology and otology, over the years, when issues arose that could have become divisive.

Returning to Northwestern as professor of audiology at the close of the war, Carhart set about immediately to develop a strong audiology graduate program and a clinical service center, placing Northwestern at the forefront in this field throughout the nation. Many of his graduates became prominent in other universities across the country as teachers, research scientists, and clinical specialists. They, as well as his many professional associates in audiology and medicine, remember him for his brilliant and inquiring mind, which provided many of the research findings still undergirding the field today; for his scholarly publications; for his masterful teaching and speaking ability; and for his skill in the management of controversial issues within his national association, now the American Speech-Language-Hearing Association. But most of all, his former students and associates remember him as a warm human being and a mentor who was first of all a friend.

Medicare) now emphasize short-term hospital stays and subsequent outpatient rehabilitative services. Audiologic services represent one form of outpatient rehabilitative service. Second, there is an increased awareness of the overall value of audiology and its contributions to health care. Finally, as was mentioned, there is a growing number of elderly individuals in the United States, with at least one-third seeking health care, including audiologic services in many cases.

Predictably, the audiologic services provided in the hospital setting tend to be medically based. These audiologic services usually focus on providing information about the identification and location of an auditory disorder. The audiologist utilizes sophisticated auditory tests to evaluate the middle ear, the inner ear, the nerve pathways to the brain, and the auditory portions of the brain. This information is then pooled with diagnostic data obtained from other disciplines, such as otology (ear specialists), neurology, pediatrics, and psychology, to derive a final diagnosis. In the hospital setting, the audiologist often works as part of a multidisciplinary team of both medical and nonmedical professionals.

Assisting the team in determining the diagnosis, however, is not the only service the audiologist provides in the hospital environment. Other services might include dispensing hearing aids, managing patients with other electronic prosthetic devices, and monitoring the hearing of patients who are treated with drugs that could damage hearing.

College and University Settings

Most major colleges and universities offer undergraduate and/or graduate training in audiology. Many audiologists with doctoral degrees assume academic positions in the university and become involved in teaching, service, and research. In order to train a clinical audiologist adequately, the university must offer appropriate clinical training experiences. Accordingly, audiologists, many without doctoral degrees, are employed by the university to service hearing-impaired patients from the community and to supervise students in training for a graduate degree in audiology. Audiologists working in this setting have frequent opportunities to participate in research and in the training of students.

Audiology in the Schools

The advent in 1975 of the Education of All Handicapped Children Act (PL 94–142), a federal law designed to assure all handicapped children a free, and appropriate public-school education, resulted in an increased awareness of the need for audiologic services in the schools. In general, the act specified that each local educational system must provide, at no cost to the child, a wide range of audiologic services. These services included hearing evaluations, auditory training, speechreading, language training, and the selection and fitting of both personal and group-type amplification units. Needless to say, such a mandate required that audiologic services be offered in the schools. Additional factors, such as the emergence of mainstreaming, have further increased the demand for educational audiology. Within the context of audiology, mainstreaming refers to the practice of placing hearing-impaired children in regular classrooms, rather than in special classrooms containing only hearing-impaired children. As more hearing-impaired children are integrated into regular classroom settings, the need to provide these children with special audiologic assistance increases. Another important variable has been the general recognition that many hearing-impaired children within the schools are not being adequately served. It has been reported, for example, that less than 50% of the hearing-impaired children in the educational system are receiving adequate services. To be sure, the introduction of PL 94–142, along with mainstreaming and an awareness of the audiologic needs of a larger group of children, has created a strong market for educational audiology. It is expected that this market will continue to grow as audiology demonstrates how significantly it can contribute to the needs of hearing-impaired children in the schools.

The responsibilities of the school audiologist include many shared by most audiologists, such as hearing screening, hearing assessment, selection and evaluation of hearing aids, and direct provision of rehabilitative services. Additional services specific to the educational setting include maintenance of personal and group hearing aids; parent counseling; in-service education to teachers, special educators, and administrators; consulting for educational placement; and serving as a liaison to the community and other professional agencies.

Audiology as a Private Practice

Certainly the fastest growing and perhaps most exciting employment setting is that of private practice. No other subgroup within the profession has shown such accelerated growth. In fact, the private practice phenomenon has created an excellent market for professional opportunities in other areas of the profession. Many audiologists are leaving the traditional employment settings attracted by the lure of a small business practice. The focus of these practices is on the sale of hearing aids. Some audiologists may operate their businesses in medical clinics, hospitals, or otolaryngology practices; others may set up their own free-standing operation. There is, of course, a substantial risk involved in setting up a small business: the Small Business Administration estimates that about 60% of all new businesses fail during the first 5 years. There are today, however, more and more successful businesses in audiology started each year.

Why is it that private practice has become so popular, and why is it growing at such a fast pace? There are several reasons. First, small businesses provide an opportunity for financial independence and entrepreneurial expression and, perhaps most importantly, an opportunity to work for oneself. Second, private practice is growing because the opportunities it provides are becoming much more visible to those audiologists working in other settings. There is a dramatic increase in the memberships of organizations that are concerned with private practice and hearing aid dispensing and in the number of publications that serve the field. We are also beginning to witness the concept of franchises or regional and national "chains" in the hearing aid dispensing business. Third, we find that the sale of hearing aids continues to increase on an annual basis and that the number of unserved hearing-impaired Americans is about 10 million, suggesting considerable potential and promise for future growth. The accelerated growth of hearing aid sales over the past several years is shown in Figure 1.2. Note that the sale of such devices remained relatively stable throughout most of the 1970s. Since 1977, however, the sale of hearing aids has been substantial, exhibiting more than a two-fold increase in less than 10 years. With the increased public awareness of hearing loss and hearing aids, the improved acoustic performance and cosmetic appeal of these instruments, and the projected increases in the number of hearing-impaired elderly, the observed growth rate in hearing aid sales is likely to continue for some time.

Community Hearing and Speech Centers

A common setting for the practice of audiology has been the community-based hearing and speech center. Today, the majority of metropolitan communities with populations greater than about 100,000 maintain community hearing and speech centers. These facilities provide comprehensive diagnostic and rehabilitative services to individuals with disorders of hearing, speech, or language. These centers receive much of their financial support from the community through individual contributions and through organizations such as the United Way and civic clubs. It is because of this type of support that such centers are able to provide services to substantial numbers of low-income patients. Audiologists are typically employed by these centers to provide a wide array of hearing services, such as hearing assessment, hearing aid selection and evaluation, hearing aid orientation, and aural rehabilitation for both hearing-impaired children and adults. Some of the larger community hearing and speech centers in the United States are also involved in conducting hearing research and in training future professionals in audiology.

Military-Based Programs

Hearing health care services are currently available in all branches of the armed forces (Army, Navy, and Air Force). As noted earlier, the military services played a key role in the historical development of the profession of audiology.

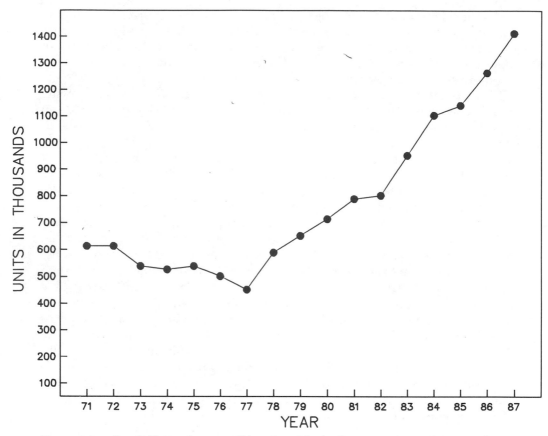

Figure 1.2.   Graph illustrating annual hearing aid sales between 1971 and 1987. (Adapted from Mahon WJ: U.S. hearing aid sales summary. *Hearing Journal* (Dec):9–13, 1988.)

In fact, immediately after World War II,'the Army set up and staffed three hospitals and the Navy, one; each of these hospitals was devoted entirely to the rehabilitation and care of military personnel with hearing impairment or other disorders of communication acquired in the military service.

An important and growing need for audiologic services still exists in the armed forces. In 1975, it was reported that as many as 50% of all service personnel exposed to combat arms suffer measurable hearing loss. Such documentation led to the recognition of a great need for military audiologists. For example, in 1967 there were only 11 audiologists employed in the Army, whereas in 1985 there were more than 70. The most dramatic change over the past several years for the employment of audiologists in the military setting has been the rapid increase in the number of female audiologists. Interestingly, it is projected that by 1992, 50% of Army audiology officers will be women. Similar changes are occurring in all other branches of the military.

The military audiologist provides a typical range of audiologic services, although there is considerable emphasis on hearing conservation, audiologic screenings and assessments, diagnostic evaluations, hearing aid evaluations, and aural rehabilitation. Military hearing conservation programs must include such components as noise measurement analysis, the use of caution signs and labels warning of hazardous exposures to noise, noise reduction measures, the selection and fitting of personal hearing protection devices, education in hearing-health care, audiometric testing, and audiologic record keeping. Finally, the military audiologist also has the opportunity to participate in research activity, primarily in the areas of aural rehabilitation and hearing conservation.

Veterans Administration Medical Centers and Other State and Federal Agencies

Most Veterans Administration (VA) medical centers maintain programs in speech-language pathology and audiology. In an effort to provide veterans with all the patient services that might be needed, the Veterans Administration has grouped medical centers into medical districts. Each medical district has a cross-section of different-sized medical centers. To receive audiologic services, the veteran typically attends the closest hospital offering an audiology program within his or her medical district.

The number of audiology and speech-language pathology programs within the VA system is growing rapidly, and this growth is expected to continue over the next several years. A recent survey revealed that between 65 and 75% of veterans exhibit significant hearing impairment. When one considers this high prevalence rate of hearing disorders, as well as the increased numbers of elderly veterans that will be expected over the next several years, it appears that the market for employment in this type of setting will be excellent.

A number of other federal agencies and state agencies also employ audiologists. At the state level, there is typically a department responsible for insuring the hearing health care needs of young children, usually associated with the Department of Public Health. Departments of public health employ audiologists to perform the full range of audiologic services and to serve as advocates for hearing-impaired children and their parents. Similarly, state departments of education and of vocational rehabilitation often employ audiologists to meet the audiologic needs of the populations their agency is charged with serving. At the federal level, most opportunities for audiologists are administrative and are not concerned with direct service delivery. Their function is usually to assist the states and regions in implementing or improving programs for hearing-handicapped citizens.

EDUCATIONAL PREPARATION FOR AUDIOLOGY

An audiologist must have a master's degree, or equivalent, in audiology from an accredited educational institution before practicing the profession. Preparation for a career in audiology, however, should begin at the undergraduate level with basic courses that will provide a strong foundation for graduate study. Courses in physics, statistics, mathematics, anatomy and physiology, psychology, child development, human behavior, and education can provide a meaningful preparation for graduate study in audiology. Students who have pursued graduate work in audiology have come from a variety of backgrounds. In a typical large graduate training program, it is not unusual to find students with a diversity of undergraduate majors, including speech-language pathology, psychology, education, and special education. Students with undergraduate majors in the basic sciences and the humanities are less frequently encountered.

It is estimated that there are over 300 colleges and universities in the United States that provide training in speech-language pathology and audiology. Of these, 118 offer master's degrees in audiology. Selecting the institution that seems to be most appropriate for a given student is sometimes difficult. Students interested in pursuing an advanced degree in audiology are encouraged to obtain the booklet, *Guide to Graduate Education in Speech-Language Pathology and Audiology*, published by the American Speech-Language-Hearing Association, one of the professional organizations for audiologists.

What is graduate training in audiology like? A graduate training profile for an audiology student enrolled in a five-semester graduate program is detailed in Vignette 1.2. Both the probable academic content of the program and the parallel practicum experiences are shown. Note that, in the first semester of study, most of the course work focuses on basic science and background information. Furthermore, the practicum during this first semester is more observation than participation. In the second semester, the introduction of the applied courses occurs, and the student becomes much more involved in practicum experiences, especially in case management. Hence, it is seen that the program progresses from basic to applied science, and that more specialization occurs during the later stages of the training program. In this example, the program offers an externship that allows the student to obtain work experience during the final semester of study. That is, a student will arrange for an 8- to 10-week practicum experience outside the university's training program. The purpose of the externship is to help the student make the transition from academic to professional life.

The master's degree is just the first step toward becoming a clinical audiologist certified by the American Speech-Language-Hearing Association (for historical reasons, generally referred to as ASHA instead of ASLHA). For the majority of audiologists, certification by ASHA is the desired clinical credential. Once the student receives the master's degree, the second step toward certification is to complete an internship known as the Clinical Fellowship Year (CFY). This means that the student must spend the first year of salaried practice under the supervision of an experienced and certified audiologist. The third step toward certification by ASHA, which can be completed at any time, is passing a national written examination in audiology.

Some students prefer to continue their graduate study and obtain the doctoral degree, most commonly the Doctor of Philosophy (Ph.D.). This program usually takes 3–4 years beyond the master's degree, and the student concentrates on theoretical and research aspects of the profession. Common employment opportunities for the Ph.D. include college and university teaching, research, and administration. Other employment settings for the doctoral level audiologist can include hospitals, clinics, and private practice.

PROFESSIONAL AFFILIATIONS

Like any professionals, audiologists should maintain affiliations with their respective professional organizations. A primary professional organization for the audiologist is the American Speech-Language-Hearing Association. As mentioned above, ASHA decides on standards of competence for the certification of

Vignette 1.2. Typical Graduate Training Profile for an Audiology Student		
Semester	Academic Content[a]	Practicum
1	*Basic science and normal background courses:* Child Development, Psychoacoustics, Physiology of Hearing, Phonetics, Psychoacoustic Instrumentation, Hearing Science, Measurement of Hearing, Research Methods	Introduction to practicum opportunities; supervised observation of diagnostic and rehabilitative techniques
2	*Case management study:* Pathologies of the Auditory System, Amplification for the Hearing Impaired I, Pediatric Audiology, Speech and Language Development	Beginning diagnostic and therapy practicum; participation in community and hospital diagnostic clinics; development of case management skills under close supervision
3	*Advanced study of communication disorders:* Speech and Language Development of Acoustically Handicapped, Language Disorders in Children, Advanced Audiologic Evaluation, Amplification for the Hearing Impaired II, Parent Counseling, Electives	Full participation in supervised diagnostic and therapy practicum; broad experience in all types of auditory disorders; introduction to private practice, schools, and hearing aid dispensing; observation and study of normal family development and educational processes; experience in parental group counseling sessions
4	*Concentration in special topics:* Seminar: Central Processing Disorders, Assistive Hearing Aid Devices, Pediatric Audiology, Medical Audiology, Auditory Electrophysiology, Aural Rehabilitation, Business Issues in Audiology	Development of independent skills in adult and child management; major responsibility for patients; written reports, professional interaction, conferences with allied professionals
5	Externship (10 weeks). Preselected sites commensurate with trainees' interests and aspirations;	Examples: (*a*) community hospital, (*b*) hospital associated with a research university, (*c*) private practice, (*d*) community hearing and speech center, (*e*) private or public schools

[a]Academic content represents topics covered during a given semester. Typically, a student will take 3–5 courses each semester.

individuals in the area of audiology (also speech-language pathology). ASHA also conducts accreditation programs for colleges and universities with degree programs in speech-language pathology and audiology and for agencies that provide clinical services to the public. Among the many services that ASHA offers its more than 50,000 members is an extensive program of continuing education. This program includes an annual national convention, national and regional conferences, institutes, and workshops. The Association also publishes professional and scientific journals, public-information material, reports and position statements, monographs, and many other special publications.

An important new professional organization for the audiologist is the American Academy of Audiology (AAA). Now comprising more than 7,000 practitioners, the profession of audiology has reached a level of size and maturity at which a need exists for a separate organization of, by, and for audiologists. With this in mind, the AAA was developed in 1988. The academy focuses on issues related to the practice of audiology, such as professional standards and ethics, publications, training, continuing education, standardization of methodologies, professional meetings, and professional scope.

Another professional affiliation for the audiologist is the American Auditory Society, an organization encompassing numerous disciplines concerned with hearing and deafness. The membership roster includes practitioners of such professions as audiology, otolaryngology, education of the hearing impaired, pediatric medicine, and psychology, as well as members of the hearing aid industry. The society sponsors an annual convention and publishes a journal, *Ear and Hearing*. The purpose of the journal is to promote conservation of hearing and to foster the habilitation and rehabilitation of the hearing impaired.

There are many other professional organizations with which the audiologist may associate, depending on the area of interest and specialization. There are professional organizations for numerous audiologic specialists including the private practitioner, the pediatric audiologist, the rehabilitative audiologist, and the audiologist employed in the academic setting.

SUMMARY

Audiology as a profession has been reviewed and discussed above. Hearing loss affects a large segment of the population of the United States, and this figure is expected to grow over the next several years. Furthermore, hearing impairment in both children and adults can be a significant handicapping condition. The profession of audiology evolved in an attempt to help the hearing impaired overcome these handicaps. Audiology has been described as a profession that is concerned with the prevention of hearing impairment and the identification, evaluation, and rehabilitation of hearing-impaired children and adults. The audiologist has numerous employment opportunities and can work in a variety of employment settings. Audiology is a young, dynamic, and challenging profession that provides a wide range of exciting opportunities for a rewarding career.

References and Suggested Readings

Bunch CC: *Clinical Audiometry*. St Louis, CV Mosby, 1943.
Cherow E: The practice of audiology—a national perspective. *ASHA* 28:31–38, 1986.
Commission on Education of the Deaf: *Toward Equality: Education of the Deaf*. A Report to the

Congress of the United States.Washington, DC, U.S. Department of Health, Education, and Welfare, 1988.

Herbst KRG: Psychosocial consequences of disorders of hearing in the elderly. In Hinchcliffe R (ed): *Hearing and Balance in the Elderly*. Edinburgh, Churchill Livingstone, 1983.

Matkin ND: Early recognition and referral of hearing impaired children. *Pediatrics in Review* 6:151–158, 1984.

Moss AJ, Parsons VL: Current estimates from the National Health Interview Survey, United States, 1985. *Vital and Health Statistics*. Series 10, no. 160. DHHS pub. no (PHS) 86–1588. Washington, DC, Public Health Services, 1986.

Northern JL, Downs MP: *Hearing in Children*, ed 3. Baltimore, Williams & Wilkins, 1984.

Sedge RK: Administration of a military-based program of speech-language pathology and audiology. In Oyer H (ed): *Administration of Programs in Speech-Language Pathology and Audiology*. Englewood Cliffs, NJ, Prentice-Hall, 1987.

Strandberg T: A national study of United States hospital speech pathology services, report number one. *ASHA* 19:69–76, 1974.

Walden B, Prosek R, Worthington D: *The Prevalence of Hearing Loss within Selected U.S. Army Branches*. Interagency No. 1A04745. Washington, DC, Army Medical Research and Development Command, 1975.

Weintraub FJ, Abeson AR, Braddock D: *State Law and Education of Handicapped Children: Issues and Recommendations*. Arlington, VA, Council for Exceptional Children, 1971.

West R: The mechanical ear. *Volta Review* 38:345–346, 1936.

CHAPTER TWO

The Nature of Sound

In this chapter, we will explore some of the fundamentals of acoustics that are essential to the understanding of audiology. The chapter begins with a discussion of selected characteristics of sound waves, which is followed by a section on the representation of sound in the time domain (its waveform) and the frequency domain (its spectrum); it concludes with a brief description of the measurement of sound.

OBJECTIVES

Following completion of this chapter, the reader should be able to:

- Describe the nature of a sound wave in terms of a series of events happening to air particles.
- Describe acoustic signals in terms of their amplitude, frequency, and phase.
- Understand the dual representation of acoustic signals in the time domain (waveform) and frequency domain (spectrum).
- Define the measure of sound level known as the decibel.

SOUND WAVES AND THEIR CHARACTERISTICS

The air we breathe is composed of millions of tiny air particles. It is the presence of these particles that makes possible the production of sound. This is made very clear by the simple yet elegant experiment described in Vignette 2.1.

It is clear from the aforementioned experiment that air particles are needed for the production and transmission of sound in the atmosphere. There are approximately 400 billion air particles in every cubic inch of the atmosphere. The billions of particles comprising the atmosphere are normally moving in a random fashion. These random continual movements of air particles are known as Brownian motion. These random movements, however, can for the most part be ignored in our discussion of sound waves. It is sufficient to assume that each particle has an average initial or resting position.

When an object surrounded by air particles vibrates, the air particles adjacent to that object also vibrate. That is, when a sufficient force is applied to the air particles by the moving object, the air particles will be moved or displaced in the

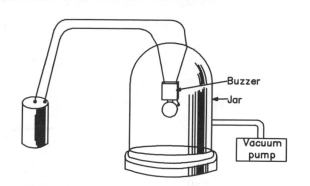

Buzzer
Jar
Vacuum pump

Vignette 2.1. The Importance of a Medium for Generating Sound

The equipment shown in the accompanying figure can be used to demonstrate the importance of air particles, or some other medium, to the generation of sound waves. An electric buzzer is placed within the jar. The jar is filled with air. When the buzzer is connected to the battery, one hears a buzzing sound originating from within the jar. Next, a vacuum is created within the jar by pumping out the air particles. When the buzzer is again connected to the battery, no sound is heard. One can see the metal components of the buzzer striking one another, yet no sound is heard. Sound waves cannot be produced without an appropriate medium, such as the air particles comprising the atmosphere.

direction of the applied force. Once the applied force is removed, a property of the air medium known as its elasticity returns the displaced particle to its resting state. The initial application of force sets up a chain of events in the surrounding air particles. This is depicted in Figure 2.1. The air particles immediately adjacent to the moving object (labeled A in Fig. 2.1) are displaced in the direction of the applied force. They then collide with more remote air particles once they have been displaced. This collision displaces the more remote particles in the direction of the applied force. The elasticity of the air returns the air particles to their resting position. As the more remote particles are colliding with air particles still further away from the vibrating object, force is applied to displace the object in the opposite direction. The void left by the former position of the object is filled by the adjacent air particles. This displaces the adjacent particle in the opposite direction. It is important to note that the vibration of air particles is passed on from one particle to another through this sequential series of collisions followed by a return to resting position. Thus, the displacement pattern produced by the object travels through the air particles via this chain of collisions. Although we could measure this vibration in particles that are a considerable distance from the source of vibration, such as the particle labeled E in Figure 2.1, each particle in the chain of collisions has only moved a very small distance and then returned to its initial position. The air particles thus form the medium through which the vibration is carried. If the air particles adjacent to the vibrating object could actually be labeled, as is done in Figure 2.1, it would be apparent that the vibration of air particles measured away from the vibrating object at point E

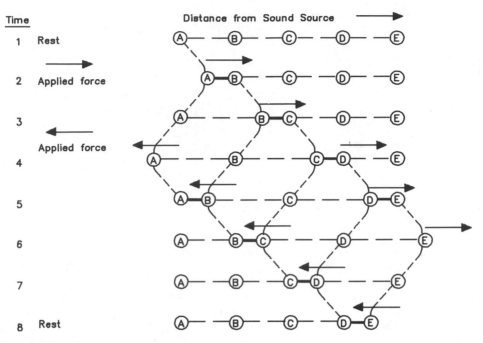

Figure 2.1. The movement of air particles (*A* through *E*) in response to an applied force at time = 2 and time = 4. The *arrows* indicate the direction of the applied force and the direction of particle displacement. Notice that each of the particles goes through a simple back-and-forth displacement. The wave propagates through the air, so that back-and-forth vibration of particle *A* eventually results in a similar back-and-forth vibration of particle *E*.

would not involve the particles next to the object, labeled *A*. Rather, the particle labeled A remains adjacent to the object at all times and simply transmits or carries the displacement from resting position to the next air particle (*B*). In turn, *B* collides with *C*, *C* with *D*, *D* with *E*, and so on. A sound wave, therefore, is the movement or propagation of a disturbance (the vibration) through a medium such as air, without permanent displacement of the particles.

Propagation of a disturbance through a medium can be demonstrated easily with the help of some friends. Six to eight persons should stand in a line, with the last person facing a wall and the others lined up behind that person. Each individual should be separated by slightly less than arm's length. Each person represents an air particle in the medium. Each individual should now place both hands firmly on the shoulders of the person immediately in front of him or her. This represents the coupling of one particle to another in the medium. Another individual should now apply some force to the medium by pushing forward on the shoulders of the first person in the chain. Note that the force applied at one end of the human chain produces a disturbance or wave that travels through the chain from one person to the next until the last person is pushed forward against the wall. The people in the chain remained in place, but the disturbance was propagated from one end of the medium to the other.

Vibration consists of movement or displacement in more than one direction.

Perhaps the most fundamental form of vibration is simple harmonic motion. Simple harmonic motion is illustrated by the pendulum in Figure 2.2. Note that the pendulum swings back and forth with the maximum displacement of *A*. The direction of displacement is indicated by the sign (+ or −) preceding the magnitude of displacement. Thus, +*A* represents the maximum displacement of the pendulum to the left, 0 represents the resting position, and −*A* represents the maximum displacement to the right. An object that vibrates in this manner in air will establish a similar back-and-forth vibration pattern in the adjacent air particles. That is, the surrounding air particles will also undergo simple harmonic motion.

The five illustrations of the pendulum on the left side of Figure 2.2 illustrate the position of the pendulum at rest and at four different instants in time. The plot in the right-hand portion of Figure 2.2 depicts the displacement as a function of time (*t*). Notice, for example, that at *t* = 0 the pendulum is displaced maximally to the left, resulting in a data point at +*A* for *t* = 0 on the graph in the right-hand portion of the figure. Similarly, at the next instant in time, *t* = 1, the pendulum returns to the resting position, or *0* displacement. This point is also

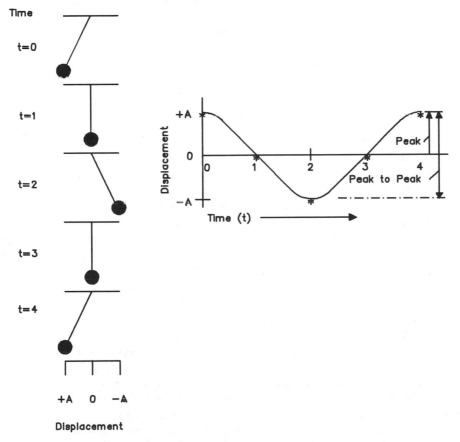

Figure 2.2. *Left*, Illustration of the movement of a pendulum at five instants in time, *t* = 0 through *t* = 4. *Right*, Notice that the simple back-and-forth vibration of the pendulum results in a sinusoidal waveform when displacement is plotted as a function of time.

plotted as an asterisk (*) in the right-hand portion of Figure 2.2. The solid line connects the displacement values produced at each moment in time. If y represents the displacement, then this *solid line* can be represented mathematically by the following equation: $y(t) = A \sin(2\pi ft + \phi)$. The details regarding this equation are not of concern here. The term t in this equation refers to various instants in time. Note that displacement and time are related to one another in this equation via the sine function. It is for this reason that simple harmonic motion is often also referred to as "sinusoidal" vibration.

All vibration, including sinusoidal vibration, can be described in terms of its amplitude (A), frequency (f), and phase (ϕ). The primary ways of expressing the amplitude or magnitude of displacement are as follows: (a) peak amplitude; (b) peak-to-peak amplitude; and (c) root-mean-square (RMS) amplitude. The latter measure of amplitude is an indicator of the average amplitude and facilitates comparisons of the amplitudes of different types of sound waves. The peak and peak-to-peak amplitudes are illustrated in the right-hand portion of Figure 2.2. Peak amplitude is the magnitude of the displacement from the resting state to the maximum amplitude. Peak-to-peak amplitude is the difference between the maximum displacement in one direction and the maximum displacement in the other direction.

The period of the vibration is the time it takes for the pendulum to move from any given point and return to the same point. This describes one complete cycle of the pendulum's movement. Notice in Figure 2.2, for example, that at $t = 4$ the pendulum has returned to the same position it occupied at $t = 0$. The period in this case would be the difference in time between $t = 0$ and $t = 4$. If each interval in time in Figure 2.2 represented one-tenth of a second (0.1 s), the period would be 0.4 s. Hence, the period may be defined as the time it takes to complete one cycle of the vibration (s/cycle).

The frequency of vibration is the number of cycles of vibration completed in one second and is measured in cycles/s. Examination of the dimensions of period (s/cycle) and frequency (cycle/s) reflects a reciprocal relationship between these two characteristics of sinusoidal vibrations. This relationship can be expressed mathematically as follows: $T = 1/f$ or $f = 1/T$, where T = period and f = frequency. Although the dimensions for frequency are cycle/s, a unit of measure defined as 1 cycle/s has been given the name *hertz*, abbreviated Hz. Thus, a sinusoidal vibration that completed one full cycle of vibration in 0.04 s (i.e., $T = 0.04$ s) would have a frequency of 25 Hz ($f = 1/T = 1$ cycle/0.04 s).

Finally, the phase (ϕ) of the vibration can be used to describe the starting position of the pendulum (starting phase) or the phase relationship between two vibrating pendulums. That is, two sinusoidal vibrations could be created that were identical in amplitude and frequency, but differed in phase, if one vibration started with the pendulum in the extreme positive position (to the left) while the other began at the extreme negative displacement (to the right). In this case, the two pendulums would be moving in opposite directions. This is called a 180° phase relationship. The two pendulums could have the same amplitude of vibration (back-and-forth movement) and move back and forth at the same rate (same frequency), yet still have different patterns of vibration.

Figure 2.3 contrasts the various features used to describe sinusoidal vibration. In Figure 2.3a, the two displacement patterns shown have identical frequen-

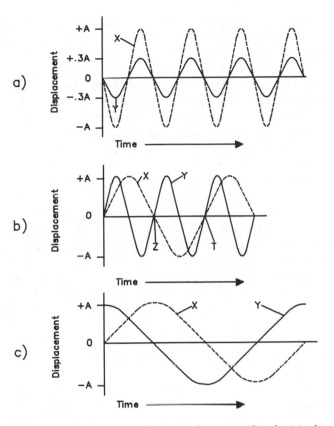

Figure 2.3. Sinusoidal waveforms differing only in amplitude (**a**), frequency (**b**), or starting phase (**c**).

cies and starting phases, but the amplitude of vibration is about three times larger for wave X. The peak amplitude of the vibration pattern labeled X is A, while that of pattern Y is 0.3A. In Figure 2.3b, on the other hand, amplitude and starting phase are equal, but the frequency of vibration for wave Y is twice as high as that for wave X. Notice, for example, that at the instant in time labeled T in Figure 2.3b, vibration pattern X has completed one full cycle of vibration, while pattern Y has completed 2 cycles at that same instant. Interestingly, note that although these two functions start in phase (both beginning at $t = 0$ with 0 displacement), their phase relationship is very complex at other instants in time. At the point labeled Z in Figure 2.3b, for example, the phase relationship is 180°. That is, at the moment in time labeled Z, both function X and Y are at 0 displacement, but one is moving in a positive direction and the other in a negative direction. Figure 2.3c illustrates two functions of identical amplitude and frequency that differ only in their starting phase. To fully describe sinusoidal vibration, all three parameters—amplitude, frequency, and starting phase—must be specified.

   In the initial discussion of the vibration of air particles, a situation was described in which force was applied to an object which resulted in the object itself displacing adjacent air particles. When the force was removed, the object and the air particles returned to their resting positions. This was a case of forced vibration. Before describing the features of forced vibration in more detail, its counterpart, free vibration, deserves brief mention. In free vibration, as in the case of the pendulum described above, once the vibration was started by applying force, the vibration continued without additional force being required to sustain it. For free vibration, the form of the vibration is always sinusoidal, and the frequency of oscillation for a particular object is always the same. This frequency is known as the object's natural or resonant frequency (Vignette 2.2). The amplitude, moreover, can be no larger than the initial displacement. If there is no resistance to oppose the sinusoidal oscillation, it will continue indefinitely. In the real world, however, this situation is never achieved. Friction opposes the vibration, which leads it to gradually decay in amplitude over time.

If one wanted to sustain the vibration or to force the object to vibrate at other than its resonant frequency, it would be necessary to apply additional force. This is forced vibration. The amplitude of displacement that results when an external or driving force is applied to the object depends, in part, on the amplitude and frequency of the applied force. For a constant amplitude of the applied force, the vibration of the object is greatest when the frequency of vibration coincides with the resonant frequency of the object. An object that vibrates maximally when a force is applied, with the stimulating frequency of the applied force corresponding to the resonant frequency of the object, is said to be at resonance. Perhaps one of the most familiar examples of acoustic resonance is the shattering of a wineglass by the high-pitched voice of a soprano. When the frequency of the applied force (the singer's voice) coincides with the natural frequency of the air-filled cavity formed by the wineglass, the maximal amplitude of vibration exceeds the maximum tolerable by the glass structure, resulting in its shattering.

Having reviewed some general features of vibration, let us now return to the discussion of sound generation and propagation. Consider the following situation. The force applied to an object surrounded by air particles is sinusoidal, resulting in a sinusoidal back-and-forth displacement of the surrounding air particles. The object displaces adjacent air particles in one direction, causing a temporary build-up or increase in density of the air particles. As the object returns to resting position due to its associated elastic restoring forces, the momentum associated with the mass of the object forces it past the resting state to its point of maximum displacement in the opposite direction. The immediately adjacent air particles attempt to fill the void left by the object, resulting in a less dense packing of air particles in this space. In so doing, the air particles surrounding the vibrating object undergo alternating periods of condensation and rarefaction. That is, the density of air particles is alternately increased and decreased relative to conditions at rest (no vibration). The increased concentration (density) of air particles results in an increase in air pressure according to a well-known law of physics, the gas law. Thus, as the vibration propagates through the air medium, a volume of atmosphere goes through alternating periods of increased and decreased air particle density and, consequently, of high and low pressure. Waves of pressure fluctuations are created and travel through the medium.

Although the pressure variations associated with sound are small compared to normal atmospheric pressure, it is these small fluctuations in pressure that are

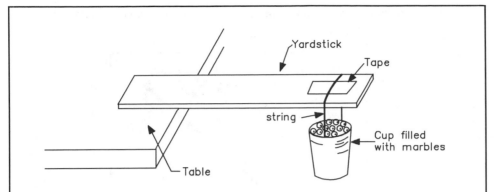

Vignette 2.2.   Conceptual Illustrations of Mass, Elasticity, and Resonance

You will be conducting a small experiment that requires the following materials: a yardstick (or meter stick), tape, 25 marbles, string (8 inches), and a small disposable cup (paper, plastic, or Styrofoam). Place the string through two small holes in the top of the cup and tie a knot at each end. Tape the string (attached to the cup) to the 1-inch mark on the yardstick. Hold or clamp 3 inches of the other end of the yardstick firmly to the top of a table. Place 5 marbles in the cup. Apply a downward force to the far end of the yardstick (the end with the cup) to bend it down approximately 2–3 inches. (Don't push down too hard or the marbles may fall out of the cup when released.) Now release the far end of the yardstick and count the number of complete up-and-down vibrations of the far end over a 5-second period. Repeat the measurements 3 times, and record the number of complete cycles of vibration during each 5-second period. This is experiment A.

Now add 20 marbles to the cup so that all 25 are now in the cup. Repeat the same procedure as above, and record the number of complete cycles three separate times. This is experiment B. If the number of complete cycles of vibration in each experiment is divided by 5 (for the 5-second measurement interval), the frequency (f) will be determined (in cycles per second). How has the system's natural frequency of vibration changed from experiment A to experiment B? By adding more marbles to the cup in experiment B, the mass of the system was increased. How was the system's natural or resonant frequency changed by increasing the mass of the system?

Now hold 12 inches of yardstick firmly against the table and repeat experiment B (25 marbles). This is experiment C. This increases the stiffness of the system. How has the resonant frequency been affected by increasing the stiffness?

The resonant frequency of an object or a medium, such as an enclosed cavity of air, is determined largely by the mass and stiffness of the object or medium. Generally, stiffness opposes low-frequency vibrations, while mass opposes high-frequency vibrations. In the figure on page 26, the opposition to vibration due to mass and stiffness is shown by the *solid lines*. The point at which these two functions cross indicates the resonant frequency of the system. The opposition to vibration due to either mass or stiffness is the lowest at this frequency. The vibration amplitude is greatest at the resonant frequency because the opposition to vibration is at its minimum value. The *dashed line* shows the effects of increasing the mass of the system. Note that the resonant frequency (the crossover point of the *dashed line* and the *solid line* representing the stiffness) has been shifted to a lower frequency. The frequency of vibration in experiment B (more mass) should have been lower than that of experiment A. In a similar manner, if stiffness is increased, the resonant frequency increases. The frequency in experiment C should have been greater than that in experiment B.

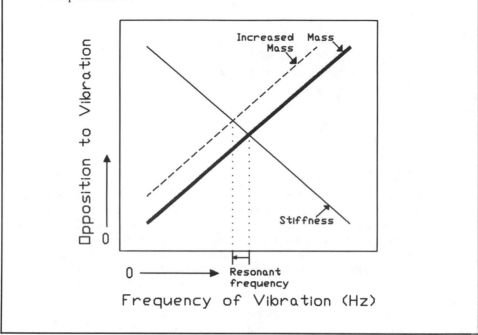

important. The pressure fluctuations, moreover, can be described using the same features discussed previously to describe changes in displacement over time. That is, a sinusoidal driving force applied to an object vibrates the object and produces sinusoidal variations in pressure. These cyclic fluctuations in pressure, moreover, can be described in terms of their amplitude, frequency, and phase. Pressure is the parameter most often used to describe sound waves because most measuring devices, such as microphones, are responsive to changes in sound pressure.

The unit of sound pressure is the pascal (abbreviated Pa). Recall that the term *hertz* rather than *cycles per second* is used to describe the frequency of a sound. The use of the term *hertz* for frequency and the term *pascal* for sound pressure reflects the contemporary practice of naming units of measure after notable scientists (Vignette 2.3). Unfortunately for the student, this practice often obscures the dimensions of the quantity. Pressure, however, is force per unit area and has frequently been described in units of either N/m^2 or d/cm^2 (N = newtons, a unit of force named after yet another famous scientist; d = dyne, a unit of force).

Although sound pressure is the preferred quantity for depicting the amplitude of a sound wave, another commonly used quantity is acoustic intensity. Acoustic intensity and sound power are used synonymously in this book. It is possible to derive the acoustic intensity corresponding to a given sound pressure. For our purposes, however, suffice it to say that acoustic intensity (I) is directly proportional to sound pressure (p) squared. That is, $I \propto p^2$.

Vignette 2.3   Units of Sound Named after Famous Scientists

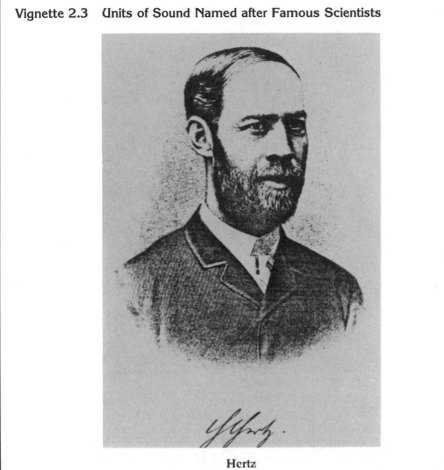

Hertz

The unit of frequency, the hertz (Hz), is named in honor of Heinrich Rudolph Hertz, a German physicist born in 1857 in Hamburg. Much of his career was devoted to the theoretical study of electromagnetic waves. This theoretical work led eventually to the development of radio, an area in which frequency is very important. Hertz died in 1894.

The sound wave propagates through air at a velocity or speed of approximately 330 m/s. This is somewhat dependent upon the characteristics of the medium, including its elasticity, density, and temperature. For example, the speed of sound in air increases with temperature from 330 m/s at 0° C to a value of 343 m/s at 20° C.

Let us suppose that a vibrating object completes one cycle of vibration when the appropriate driving force is applied. As the first condensation of air particles, or local high-pressure area, is created, it travels away from the source. At the completion of one cycle, a new high-pressure area is created. By the time a second high-pressure area is completed, however, the first has traveled still

Vignette 2.3   (Continued)

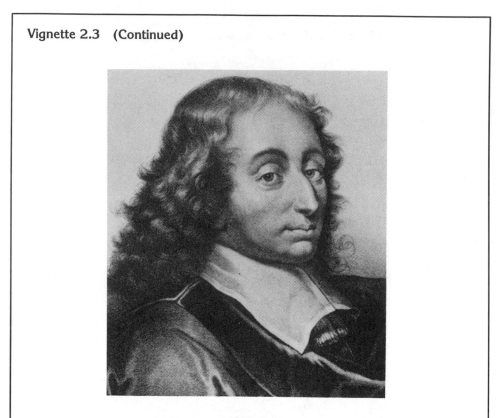

Pascal

   The unit of sound pressure, the pascal (Pa), is named in honor of Blaise Pascal (1623–1662). Pascal was a French scientist and philosopher. He is well known for his contributions to both fields. As a scientist, he was both a physicist and a mathematician. In 1648, Pascal proved empirically that the mercury column in a barometer is affected by atmospheric pressure and not a vacuum, as previously believed. Thus, his name is linked in history with research concerning the measurement of atmospheric pressure.

further from its point of origin. The distance between these two successive condensations or high-pressure areas is called the wavelength of the sound wave. Now if the frequency of vibration is high, the separation between successive high-pressure areas is small. Recall that a high frequency implies a short period ($f = 1/T$). That is, the time it takes for one complete cycle is short for high frequencies. Consequently, the first high-pressure area is unable to travel far from the source before the second high-pressure area arises. Thus, the wavelength (λ), the separation in distance between successive high-pressure areas, is small. The wavelength (λ), frequency (f), and speed of sound (c) are related in the following manner: $\lambda = c/f$. Wavelength varies inversely with frequency; the higher the frequency, the shorter the wavelength.

   To clarify the concept of wavelength and its inverse relationship to frequency, consider once again the human chain that represented adjacent air

---

Vignette 2.3   (Continued)

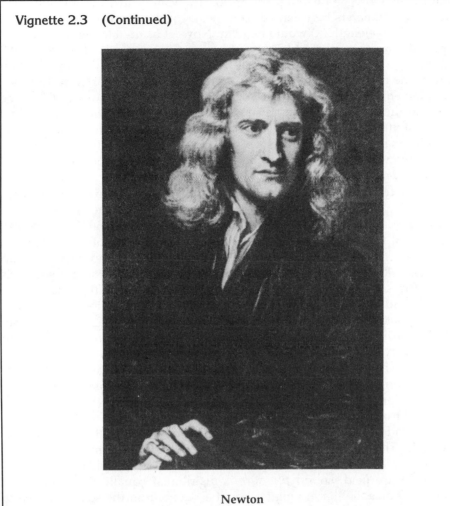

Newton

The newton (N), the unit of force, is named in honor of the well-known English mathematician, physicist, and astronomer Sir Isaac Newton (1642–1727), who spent much of his career studying various aspects of force. Of his many discoveries and theories, perhaps the two best known are his investigations of gravitational forces and his three laws of motion.

---

particles. Suppose that, once a force was applied to the shoulders of the first person, it took 10 seconds for the disturbance (the push) to travel all the way to the end of the human chain. Let us also say that the chain had a length of 10 m. If a force was applied to the shoulders of the first person every 10 seconds, the frequency of vibration would be 0.1 Hz ($f = 1/T = 1/10$ s). Moreover, 10 seconds after the first push, the second push would be applied. Because we have stated that 10 seconds would be required for the disturbance to travel to the last person in the chain, when the second push is applied, the last person in the chain (10 m away) would also be pushing forward on the wall. Thus, there would be a separation of 10 meters between adjacent peaks of the disturbance or forward pushes. The wavelength (λ) would be 10 m. Now let us double the frequency of the applied force to a value of 0.2 Hz. The period is 5 seconds ($T = 1/f = 1/0.2 = 5$ s). Every 5 seconds, a new force will be applied to the shoulders of the first person in the chain. Because it takes 10 seconds for the disturbance to travel through the entire 10-m chain, after 5 seconds the first disturbance will only be 5 m away as the second push is applied to the shoulders of the first person. Thus, the wavelength, or the separation between adjacent "pushes" in the medium, is 5 m. Notice that when the frequency of the applied force was doubled from 0.1 to 0.2 Hz, the wavelength was halved from 10 m to 5 m. Frequency and wavelength are inversely related.

Another feature of sound waves that is obvious to almost anyone with normal hearing is that the sound pressure decreases in amplitude as the distance it travels increases. Under special measurement conditions, in which sound waves are not reflected from surrounding surfaces and the sound source is a special source, known as a point source, the decrease in sound pressure with distance is well defined. Specifically, as the distance from the sound source is doubled, the sound pressure is halved. Similarly, based on the relationship between sound pressure and acoustic intensity described previously ($I \propto p^2$), it is apparent that the same doubling of distance would reduce the acoustic intensity to $\frac{1}{4}$ [$(\frac{1}{2})^2$] the initial value. This well-defined dependence of sound pressure and sound intensity on distance is known as the inverse square law.

So far, we have considered some of the characteristics or features of a single sound wave originating from one source. Moreover, we have assumed that the sound wave was propagating through a special environment in which the wave is not reflected from surrounding surfaces. This type of environment, one without reflected sound waves, is known as a free field. A diffuse field is the complement of a free field. That is, in a diffuse field, sound is reflected from many surfaces. The inverse square law that was just described holds only for free-field conditions. In fact, in a diffuse field, sound pressure is distributed equally throughout the measurement area, so that no matter how far we go from the sound source or where we are in the measurement area, the sound pressure is the same. The term sound field is sometimes used to describe a region containing sound waves. Free fields and diffuse fields, then, are special classes of sound field.

Interference results when two sound waves encounter one another. The two sound waves referred to here may be two independent waves arising from separate sources (e.g., two loudspeakers) or the original wave (usually called the incident sound wave) and its reflection off a wall, ceiling, floor, or other surface. The interference that results when two sound waves encounter one another may be either constructive or destructive. In constructive interference, the two sound waves add together to yield a resulting sound wave that is greater in amplitude than either wave alone. This is illustrated in the left-hand portion of Figure 2.4. In the case shown here, in which both waves are of equal amplitude, the maximum possible constructive interference would be a doubling of amplitude. Negative interference, on the other hand, occurs whenever the amplitude of the sound wave resulting from the interaction is less than the amplitude of either wave

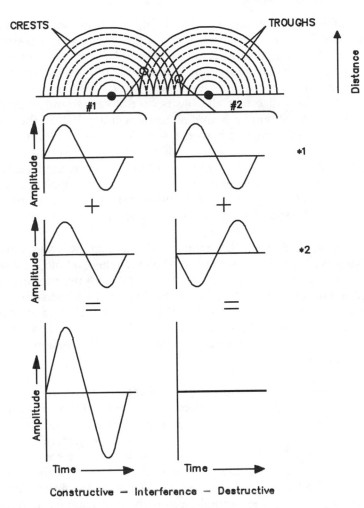

Figure 2.4. Illustration of constructive and destructive interference of two sound waves (#1 and #2). The origin of each wave is represented by the *black circles* in the upper portion of the figure. The graph at the *lower left* illustrates the combination of waves #1 and #2 when the crests of each wave coincide. The two waves are in phase at this point, and the resulting sound wave is greater than either wave alone. This is constructive interference. The graph at the *lower right* illustrates the combination of the crest of wave #1 and the trough of wave #2. The two waves are 180° out of phase at this point, resulting in a complete cancellation of the two waves. This is destructive interference. (Adapted from Durrant JD, Lovrinic JH: *Bases of Hearing Science*, ed 2. Baltimore, Williams & Wilkins, 1986, p 41).

alone. The extreme case of negative interference results in the complete cancellation of the sound waves, as illustrated in the right-hand portion of Figure 2.4.

In addition to the interference that results when two sound waves interact, there are other interference effects that result when a sound wave encounters an object or structure of some kind. When a sound wave encounters an object, the outcome of this encounter is determined in large part by the dimensions and composition of the object and the wavelength of the sound. When the dimensions of the object are large relative to the wavelength of the sound wave, a sound shadow results. This is analogous to the more familiar light shadow in which an object in the path of light casts a shadow behind it. In the case of a sound shadow, the object creates an area without sound, or a "dead area," immediately behind it. It is important to realize that all objects do not cast sound shadows for all sound waves. The creation of a sound shadow will depend on the dimensions of the object and the wavelength of the sound. For example, a cube having dimensions of 1 m × 1 m × 1 m, will not cast a shadow for sound waves having a wavelength that is much larger than 1 m. Recall that wavelength and frequency vary inversely. In this example, a sound wave having a wavelength of 1 m has a frequency of 330 Hz ($f = c/\lambda$; $c = 330$ m/s; $\lambda = 1$ m). Thus, the object in this example would cast a sound shadow for frequencies greater than 330 Hz ($\lambda < 1$ m).

Finally, let us consider what happens when a sound wave encounters a barrier of some type. First, let us consider the case where a hole is present in the barrier. In this case, as was the case for the sound shadow, the results depend on the wavelength (and, therefore, frequency) of the incident sound wave and the dimensions of the hole. For wavelengths much greater than the dimensions of the hole, the sound wave becomes diffracted. Diffraction is a change in direction of the sound wave. Thus, under these conditions the direction of the incident sound wave can be altered.

If the sound wave encounters a barrier that contains no holes, varying degrees of sound transmission, absorption, or reflection can occur. The proportion of the sound wave's energy reflected by the barrier and the proportion transmitted through the barrier depend on the similarity of the barrier's and the medium's impedance. Impedance may be thought of very generally as opposition to the flow of energy, in this case the advancement of the sound wave. If the barrier and the medium have the same impedance, 100% of the energy of the sound wave will be transmitted through the barrier. If the difference in impedances, often referred to as the "impedance mismatch," is large, then most of the incident sound wave will be reflected and little will be transmitted across the barrier (Vignette 2.4).

Aside from being reflected or transmitted, a portion of the sound wave may also be absorbed by the barrier. In the absorption of sound energy, the acoustic energy of the impinging sound wave is changed to heat. The materials out of which the barrier is constructed determine its ability to absorb sound.

WAVEFORMS AND THEIR ASSOCIATED SPECTRA

Many of the important features of a sound wave, such as its amplitude, period, and frequency, can be summarized in either of two common formats. One format, the waveform, describes the acoustic signal in terms of amplitude variations as a function of time. The sinusoidal waveform described previously for simple harmonic motion is an example of a waveform or time-domain representation of an acoustic signal. For every waveform, there is an associated representation of that signal in the frequency domain, called the amplitude and phase spectrum. Figure 2.5a illustrates the amplitude and phase spectrum for a simple sinusoidal waveform. Note that the x axis of the spectrum is frequency, while

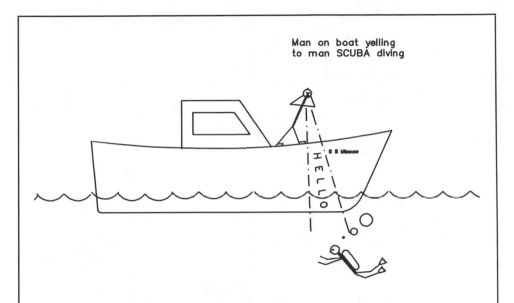

Man on boat yelling
to man SCUBA diving

Vignette 2.4.   Discussion of Impedance Mismatch between Air and Water

Consider the following situation. You and a friend are out on a boat in the ocean, scuba diving. Your friend is already underwater and you want to talk to him. He's only a few feet below the surface, yet, despite your yelling, he doesn't respond. Why not? The sound waves carrying your voice are travelling through an air medium. When the sound waves encounter the surface of the ocean water, a change in impedance is encountered. The impedance of ocean water is a few thousand times greater than that of air. As a consequence, only about 0.1% of the sound energy will be transmitted beneath the surface of the water to your friend. Approximately 99.9% of the airborne sound wave is reflected away from the surface. Thus, the impedance mismatch between the air and ocean water results in almost all of the airborne sound energy being reflected away from the surface.

the y axis is either amplitude or phase. The amplitude scale can be peak-to-peak amplitude, peak amplitude, or RMS amplitude, as described previously. The phase spectrum in this case illustrates the starting phase of the acoustic signal. There can only be one possible waveform associated with the amplitude and phase spectrum shown in the right-hand side of Figure 2.5a. Similarly, there is only one set of amplitude and phase spectra associated with the waveform in the left-hand side of Figure 2.5a. Thus, both the time-domain and frequency-domain representation of the acoustic stimulus uniquely summarize its features. Furthermore, knowing one, we can derive the other. For every waveform, there is one and only one amplitude spectrum and phase spectrum associated with it. For every amplitude and phase spectrum, there is one and only one possible waveform.

Simple sinusoidal sounds are more the exception than the rule in everyday encounters with sound. Over a century ago, however, a mathematician named Fourier determined that all complex periodic sounds consisted of a sum of simple

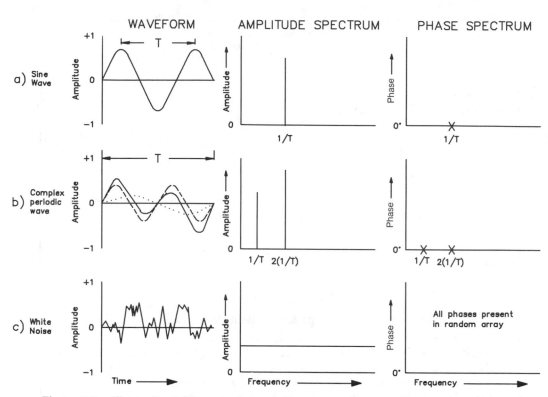

Figure 2.5. Illustration of the waveforms and corresponding amplitude and phase spectra for a continuous sine wave (**a**); a complex periodic wave (**b**) (*solid line* is complex waveform, *dashed* and *dotted lines* are the two sine waves making up the complex sound); and white noise (**c**).

sinusoids. A periodic sound is one in which the waveform repeats itself every T seconds. In the left-hand portion of Figure 2.5**b**, a complex periodic waveform is illustrated by the *solid line*. The *dashed* and *dotted waveforms* illustrate the two sinusoidal signals that, when added together, yield the complex sound. The spectrum of the complex sound then can be represented by the sum of the spectra of both sinusoidal components. This is illustrated in the right-hand portion of Figure 2.5**b**. Complex periodic sounds, such as that shown in Figure 2.5**b**, have a special type of amplitude spectra known as line spectra. That is, the amplitude spectrum consists of a series of discrete lines located at various frequencies and having specified amplitudes. Each line represents a separate sinusoidal component of the complex sound. The component having the lowest frequency is called the fundamental frequency. The fundamental frequency corresponds to $1/T$, where T is the period of the complex sound. Additional components located at frequencies corresponding to integer multiples of the fundamental frequency are referred to as harmonics of the fundamental. If the fundamental frequency is 200 Hz, for example, the second and third harmonics of 200 Hz are 400 Hz (2 × 200 Hz) and 600 Hz (3 × 200 Hz), respectively. The first harmonic corresponds to the fundamental frequency. Additionally, the term octave means a doubling of frequency. Continuing the same example, 400 Hz would lie 1 octave above the fundamental frequency (200 Hz), while 800 Hz would be 2 octaves (another doubling) above the fundamental frequency.

Many acoustic signals in our environment are not periodic. Noise is probably the most common example. Noise is said to be an aperiodic signal because it fails to repeat itself at regular intervals. Rather, the waveform for noise shows amplitude varying randomly over time. This is illustrated in the left-hand portion of Figure 2.5c. The case shown here is an example of a special type of noise called white noise. White noise is characterized by an average amplitude spectrum that has uniform amplitude across frequency. That is, there is equal sound energy at all frequencies. This is depicted in the right-hand portion of Figure 2.5c. Note that the amplitude spectrum no longer consists of a series of lines. Rather, a continuous function is drawn which reflects equal amplitude at all frequencies. Aperiodic waveforms, such as noise, have continuous amplitude spectra, not discrete line spectra.

A variety of noises can be obtained from white noise using devices known as filters. Filters are typically electronic devices that selectively pass energy in some frequency regions and block the passage of energy at other frequencies. If we begin with white noise, an acoustic signal having energy at all frequencies, and send that noise through a filter called a low-pass filter, which passes only the low frequencies, the result is a low-pass noise that contains equal amplitude at low frequencies and little or no sound energy at high frequencies. A low-pass filter passes the low frequencies and filters out the high frequencies. In a similar manner, other noises, such as high-pass noise (sound energy at high frequencies only), can be generated. It should be noted that filters can be applied to a variety of acoustic signals, not just noise, to eliminate energy in certain frequency regions.

It has already been indicated that it is possible to represent an acoustic signal in both the frequency domain and the time domain. So far in our discussion of waveforms and spectra, it has been assumed that the acoustic signals are continuous (≥ 1 s). Often, however, this is not the case. As a general rule, the shorter the duration of the signal, the broader the amplitude spectrum. Thus, a 1000-Hz pure tone that is turned on, and then turned off 0.1 second later, will have sound energy at several frequencies other than 1000 Hz. Approximately 90% of the sound energy will fall between 990 and 1010 Hz. If the duration of the pure tone is decreased to 0.01 second, 90% of the sound energy will be distributed from 900 through 1100 Hz. Hence, as the duration decreases, the spread of sound energy to other frequencies increases. The limit to the decrease in duration would be an infinitely short pulse or click-like sound. For this hypothetical sound, energy would spread equally to all frequencies.

SOUND MEASUREMENT

As mentioned previously, the amplitude of a sound wave is typically expressed as sound pressure (p) in units of pascals (Pa). Recall that one of the major reasons for this was that most measuring devices are pressure detectors. That is, devices such as microphones are sensitive to variations in air pressure and convert these pressure variations to variations in electrical voltage. In more general terms, the microphone can be referred to as an acousticoelectrical transducer. A transducer is any device that changes energy from one form to another. In this case, the conversion is from acoustical to electrical energy.

Although the overall amplitude of sound waves is best expressed in terms of RMS pressure, the use of the actual physical units to describe the level of sound is cumbersome. In humans, the ratio of the highest tolerable sound pressure to the sound pressure that can just be heard exceeds 10,000,000:1! Moreover, the units dictate that one would be dealing frequently with numbers much smaller than 1. The lowest sound pressure that can just be heard by an average young adult with normal hearing, for instance, is approximately 0.00002 Pa (or 2×10^{-5} Pa; 20 μPa).

Rather than deal with this cumbersome system based on the physical units of pressure, scientists devised a scale known as the decibel scale. The decibel scale quantifies the sound level by taking the logarithm (base 10) of the ratio of two sound pressures and multiplying it by 20. That is, the following formula is used to calculate the sound level in decibels (dB) from the ratio of two sound pressures (p_1 and p_2): $20 \log_{10} (p_1/p_2)$. Let us again use the range of sound pressures from maximum tolerable to just audible (10,000,000:1) to see how this range would be represented in decibels. To do this, we begin by substituting 10,000,000/ 1 for p_1/p_2. The $\log_{10}$ of 10,000,000 (or 10^7) is 7. When 7 is multiplied by 20, the result is 140 dB. We have taken a scale represented by a range of physical sound pressures of 10,000,000:1 and compressed it to a much more manageable range of 0 to 140 dB. The greatest sound pressure that can be tolerated is 140 dB greater than the sound pressure that can barely be detected.

Notice that the preceding statement only indicates that the sound pressure that is just tolerable is 140 dB above that which can just be heard, but does not indicate what either of those sound pressures is in units of Pa. This is because a ratio of two sound pressures has been used in the calculation of dB, and ratios are dimensionless quantities. That is, we are calculating the decibel increase of one sound relative to another. Sometimes all we are interested in is a relative change in sound pressure. Recall from the discussion of the inverse square law, for example, that as distance doubled from the sound source, the sound pressure was halved. The corresponding change in decibels associated with this halving of sound pressure can be calculated by using a ratio of 0.5/1. The $\log_{10}$ of 0.5 is $-.301$, which, when multiplied by 20, yields a change in sound pressure of approximately -6 dB. We can restate the inverse square law by indicating that as the distance from the sound source is doubled, the sound pressure decreases by 6 dB. Again, this does not indicate what the values are of the two sound pressures involved in this change. The sound pressure may begin at 10 Pa and be halved to 5 Pa or may start at 10,000 Pa and decrease to 5,000 Pa. Either of these cases corresponds to a halving of the initial sound pressure which corresponds to a 6-dB decrease.

Often, an indication of the sound pressure level is needed that provides an absolute rather than a relative indication of the sound level. To accomplish this, it is necessary to evaluate all sound pressures relative to the same reference sound pressure. That is, the denominator of the decibel equation becomes a fixed value called the reference sound pressure. The reference sound pressure for a scale known as the sound pressure level (SPL) scale is 2×10^{-5} Pa. As noted above, this corresponds to the softest sound pressure that can be heard by humans under optimal conditions. Calculation of the sound pressure level (*SPL*) for a specific sound pressure (p_1) can be accomplished by solving the following equation: *SPL* in dB $= 20 \log [p_1/(2 \times 10^{-5}$ Pa)]. Perhaps the simplest case to consider is the lowest sound pressure that can just be heard, i.e., 2×10^{-5} Pa. If $p_1 = 2 \times 10^{-5}$ Pa, then the ratio formed by the two sound pressures is $(2 \times 10^{-5}$ Pa)/$(2 \times 10^{-5}$ Pa), or 1. The log of 1 is 0, which, when multiplied by 20, yields a sound level of 0 dB SPL. Consequently, 0 dB SPL does not mean absence of sound. Rather, it simply corresponds to a sound pressure of 2×10^{-5} Pa. Sound pressures lower than this value will yield negative SPL values, while sound pressures greater than this yield positive values.

Let us consider another example. A sound pressure of 1 Pa corresponds to how many dB SPL? This can be restated by asking the reader to solve the following: *SPL* in dB $= 20 \log [1.0$ Pa/$(2 \times 10^{-5}$ Pa)]. We begin by first reducing $1.0/(2 \times 10^{-5})$ to 5×10^4. The log of 5×10^4 is approximately 4.7, which, when multiplied by 20, yields a sound pressure level of 94 dB. Thus, a sound pressure of 1 Pa yields a sound pressure level of 94 dB SPL. This sound level is within the range of typical noise levels encountered in many factories.

Fortunately, laborious calculations are not required every time measurements of sound pressure level are required. Rather, simple devices have been constructed to measure the level of various acoustic signals in dB SPL. These devices, known as sound level meters, utilize a microphone to change the sound pressure variations to voltage variations. The RMS amplitude of these voltage variations is then determined within the electronic circuitry of the meter, and an indicator (needle or pointer, digital display, etc.) responds accordingly. In the case of 1 Pa RMS sound pressure input to the microphone, for example, the meter would either point to or display a value of 94 dB SPL.

Other measuring devices may be used to measure other features of the sound waves. Filters, for example, can be used in conjunction with the sound level meter to determine the amplitude of various frequencies contained in a sound. One can get at least a gross estimate of the amplitude spectrum of an acoustic signal by successively examining adjacent frequency regions of the signal. This can be accomplished with filters. For example, the filter might first be set to pass only low frequencies and the sound pressure level measured with the sound level meter. The filter could then be adjusted so as to pass only intermediate frequencies, then high frequencies, and so forth. This would provide a gross indication of how much sound energy was contained in various frequency regions. Very detailed and fine descriptions of the amplitude spectrum could be obtained by using narrow filters or by using a device known as a spectrum analyzer. The latter device essentially provides a plot of the amplitude spectrum associated with the waveform. The waveform itself may be examined in detail through the use of a device known as an oscilloscope. An oscilloscope displays the waveform of the sound impinging on the microphone. Various means can be used to either "freeze" or store the waveform until all of its details (amplitude, period, phase, etc.) have been quantified.

Microphones, sound level meters, electronic filters, spectrum analyzers, and oscilloscopes represent just a few of the basic tools utilized by the scientist and the clinician in the measurement of sound. The audiologist frequently uses these tools to check the equipment used in the testing of hearing. This equipment must be checked frequently to ensure that the results obtained with the equipment are accurate and that other clinics could obtain the same findings from a given patient.

SUMMARY

The fundamentals of acoustics were reviewed in this chapter. Simple harmonic motion, or sinusoidal vibration, was discussed. The effects of varying the amplitude, frequency, and starting phase of the sinusoidal waveform were examined. The relation between the representations of sound in the time domain, the waveform, and sound in the frequency domain, the amplitude and phase spectra, were reviewed. A discussion of resonance and its relation to impedance was also included. Finally, the measurement of sound levels in decibels (dB) was reviewed.

References and Suggested Readings

Beranek LL: *Acoustics*. New York, McGraw-Hill, 1954.
Berlin CI: *Programmed Instruction on the Decibel*. Kresge Hearing Research Laboratory of the South, Louisiana State University School of Medicine, 1970.
Cudahy E: *Introduction to Instrumentation in Speech and Hearing*. Baltimore, Williams & Wilkins, 1988.
Denes PB, Pinson EN: *The Speech Chain*. New York, Bell Telephone Laboratories, 1963.
Durrant JD, Lovrinic JH: *Bases of Hearing Science*, ed 2. Baltimore, Williams & Wilkins, 1984.
Small AM: *Elements of Hearing Science: A Programmed Text*. New York, John Wiley & Sons, 1978.
Yost WA, Nielsen DW: *Fundamentals of Hearing: An Introduction*. New York, Holt, Rinehart, & Winston, 1985.

CHAPTER THREE

Structure and Function of the Auditory System

This chapter is divided into three main sections. The first two deal with the anatomy, physiology, and functional significance of the peripheral and central sections of the auditory system. The peripheral portion of the auditory system is defined here as the structures from the outer ear through the auditory nerve. The central auditory nervous system begins at the cochlear nucleus and is bounded at the other end by the auditory centers of the cortex. The third section of this chapter details some fundamental aspects of the perception of sound.

OBJECTIVES

Following completion of this chapter, the reader should be able to:

- Recognize and identify some key anatomic features or landmarks of the auditory system.
- Understand the functional roles of the outer ear and middle ear.
- Understand the mapping of frequency to place (tonotopic organization) that occurs throughout the auditory system.
- Recognize the ability of the peripheral auditory system to code information in both a time-domain and frequency-domain representation.
- Appreciate some basic auditory perceptual phenomena, such as loudness and masking.

PERIPHERAL AUDITORY SYSTEM

Figure 3.1 shows a cross-section of the peripheral portion of the auditory system. This portion of the auditory system is usually further subdivided into the outer ear, middle ear, and inner ear.

Outer Ear

The outer ear consists of two primary components: the pinna and the ear canal. The pinna is the most visible portion of the ear, which extends laterally from the side of the head. It is composed of cartilage and skin. The ear canal is the long, narrow canal leading to the eardrum. The entrance to this canal is called

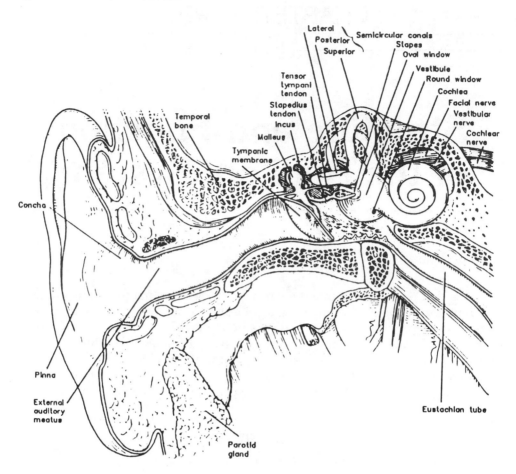

Figure 3.1.   A cross section of the peripheral portion of the auditory system revealing some of the anatomic details of the outer, middle, and inner ear. (Adapted from Kessel, RG and Kardon, RH *Tissues and Organs: A Text-Atlas of Scanning Electron Microscopy.* W. H. Freeman and Co. San Francisco, 1979)

the external auditory meatus. The deep bowl-like portion of the pinna adjacent to the external auditory meatus is known as the concha.

   The outer ear serves a variety of functions. First, the long (2.5-cm), narrow (5- to 7-mm) canal makes the more delicate middle and inner ear less accessible to foreign bodies. The outer third of the canal, moreover, is composed of skin and cartilage lined with glands and hairs. These glands, known as ceruminous glands, secrete a substance that potential intruders, such as insects, find to be terribly noxious. So both the long, narrow, tortuous path of the canal and the secretions of these glands serve to protect the remaining portions of the peripheral auditory system.

   Second, the various air-filled cavities comprising the outer ear, the two most prominent being the concha and the ear canal, have a natural or resonant frequency to which they respond best. This is true of all air-filled cavities. For the ear canal of the adult, the resonant frequency is approximately 2500 Hz, while that of the concha is roughly 5000 Hz. The resonance of each of these cavities is such that each structure increases the sound pressure at its resonant frequency by about 10–12 dB. This gain or increase in sound pressure provided by the outer ear can best be illustrated by considering the following hypothetical experiment. Let us begin by using two tiny microphones. One microphone will be placed just outside (lateral to) the concha, and the other will be positioned very carefully inside the ear canal so as to rest alongside the eardrum. Now if we present a series of sinusoidal sound waves, or pure tones, of different frequencies, which all measure 70 dB SPL at the microphone just outside the concha, and if we read the sound pressure levels measured with the other microphone near the eardrum, we will obtain results like those shown by the *solid line* in Figure 3.2. Notice that, at frequencies less than approximately 1400 Hz, the microphone located near the eardrum measures sound levels of approximately 73 dB SPL. This is only 3 dB higher than the sound level just outside the outer ear. Consequently, the outer ear exerts little effect on the intensity of low-frequency sound. The intensity of the sound measured at the eardrum increases to levels considerably above 70 dB SPL, however, as the frequency of the sound is increased. The maximum sound level at the eardrum is reached at approximately 2500 Hz and corresponds to a value of approximately 87 dB SPL. Thus, when sound waves having a frequency of 2500 Hz enter the outer ear, their sound pressure is increased by 17 dB by the time they strike the eardrum. The

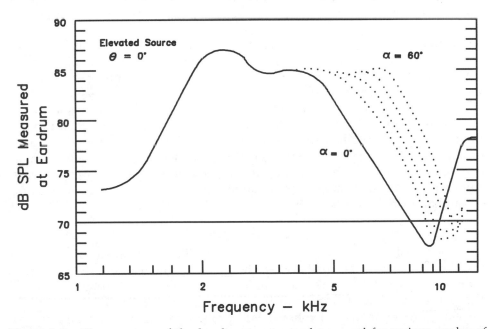

Figure 3.2. The response of the head, outer ear, and ear canal for various angles of elevation (α) of the sound source. Zero degrees corresponds to a sound source at eye level and straight ahead (0° azimuth, Θ) while 60° represents a source located straight ahead but at a higher elevation. If the listener's head and outer ear had no influence on the sound level measured at the eardrum, a flat line at 70 dB SPL would result. This figure illustrates the amplification of high-frequency sound by the outer ear and the way that this amplification pattern changes with elevation of the sound source. (Adapted from Shaw EAG: The external ear. In Keidel WD, Neff WD (eds): *Handbook of Sensory Physiology*. New York, Springer Verlag, 1974, vol 5(1), p 463.)

function drawn with a *solid line* in Figure 3.2 illustrates the role that the outer ear serves as a resonator or amplifier of high-frequency sounds. The function shown is for the entire outer ear. Experiments similar to the one just described can be conducted to isolate the contribution of various cavities to the resonance of the total outer ear system. Again, the results of such experiments suggest that the two primary structures contributing to the resonance of the outer ear are the concha and the ear canal.

The resonance of the outer ear which is represented by the *solid line* in Figure 3.2 was obtained with a sound source located directly in front of the subject at eye level. If the sound source is elevated by varying amounts, a different resonance curve is obtained. Specifically, the notch or dip in the solid function that is located at 10 kHz in Figure 3.2 moves to a higher frequency and the peak of the resonant curve broadens to encompass a wider range of frequencies as the sound source is increased in elevation. This is illustrated in Figure 3.2 by the *dotted lines.* Each dotted line represents a different angle of elevation. An elevation of 0° corresponds to eye level, while 90° elevation would position the sound source directly overhead. The response of the outer ear changes as the elevation of the sound source changes. This results from the angle at which the incident sound wave strikes the various cavities of the outer ear. The result is that a code for sound elevation is provided by the outer ear. This code is the amplitude spectrum of the sound, especially above 3000 Hz, that strikes the eardrum. Thus, the outer ear plays an important role in the perception of the elevation of a sound source.

Finally, the outer ear also assists in another aspect of the localization of a sound source. The orientation of the pinnae is such that the pinnae collect sound more efficiently from sound sources located in front of the listener than from sources originating behind the listener. The attenuation of sound waves originating from behind the listener assists in the front/back localization of sound.

In summary, the outer ear serves four primary functions. First, it protects the more delicate middle and inner ears from foreign bodies. Second, it boosts or amplifies high-frequency sounds. Third, the outer ear provides the primary cue for the determination of the elevation of a sound's source. Fourth, the outer ear assists in distinguishing sounds that arise from in front of the listener from those that arise from behind the listener.

Middle Ear

The middle ear consists of a small (2-cm^3) air-filled cavity lined with a mucous membrane. It forms the link between the air-filled outer ear and the fluid-filled inner ear (Fig. 3.1). This link is accomplished mechanically via three tiny bones, the ossicles. The lateralmost ossicle is the malleus. The malleus is in contact with the eardrum or tympanic membrane. At the other end of the outer ear/inner ear link is the smallest, medialmost ossicle, the stapes. The broad base of the stapes, known as the footplate, rests in a membranous covering of the fluid-filled inner ear referred to as the oval window. The middle ossicle in the link, sandwiched between the malleus and stapes, is the incus. The ossicles are suspended loosely within the middle ear by ligaments, known as the axial ligaments, extending from the anterior and posterior walls of the cavity. There are other connections between the surrounding walls of the middle ear cavity and the ossicles. Two connections are formed by the small middle ear muscles, the tensor tympani and the stapedius. The tensor tympani originates from the anterior (front) wall of the cavity and attaches to a region of the malleus called the neck, while the stapedius has its origin in the posterior (back) wall of the tympanic cavity and inserts near the neck of the stapes.

We have mentioned that the middle ear cavity is air filled. The air filling the cavity is supplied via a tube that connects the middle ear to the upper part of the throat, or the nasopharynx. This tube, known as the auditory tube or the eustachian tube, has one opening located along the bottom of the anterior wall of the middle ear cavity. The tube is normally closed but can be readily opened by yawning or swallowing. In adults, the eustachian tube assumes a slight downward orientation. This facilitates drainage of fluids from the middle ear cavity into the nasopharynx. Thus, the eustachian tube serves two primary purposes. First, it supplies air to the middle ear cavity and thereby enables an equalization of the air pressure on both sides of the eardrum. This is desirable for efficient vibration of the eardrum. Second, the eustachian tube permits the drainage of fluids from the middle ear into the nasopharynx.

What is the purpose of the elaborate link between the air-filled outer ear and the fluid-filled inner ear formed by the three ossicles? Recall from the example in Chapter 2 that the barrier formed by the interface between the media of air and sea water resulted in a "loss" of approximately 99.9% of the sound energy. That is, 99.9% of the energy in the impinging sound wave was reflected away, and only 0.1% was transmitted into the water. This loss amounts to a decrease in sound energy of approximately 30 dB. If the middle ear did not exist, and the membranous entrance of the fluid-filled inner ear (oval window) replaced the eardrum, sound waves carried in air would impinge directly on the fluid-filled inner ear. This barrier is analogous to the air-to-water interface described above. Consequently, if such an arrangement existed, there would be a considerable loss of sound energy.

The middle ear compensates for this loss of sound energy when going from air to a fluid medium through two primary mechanisms. The first of these, the areal ratio (ratio of the areas) of the tympanic membrane to the footplate of the stapes, accounts for the largest portion of the compensation. The effective area of the tympanic membrane, i.e., the area involved directly in the mechanical link between the outer ear and inner ear, is approximately 55 mm^2. The corresponding area of the stapes footplate is 3.2 mm^2. Pressure (p) may be defined in terms of force (F) per unit area (A) ($p=F/A$). If the force applied at the eardrum is the same as that reaching the stapes footplate, then the pressure at the smaller footplate must be greater than that at the larger eardrum. That is, given $F_1=F_2$, $F_1/3.2 > F_2/55$. The ratio of these two areas is 55/3.2=17. Consequently, the pressure at the oval window is 17 times greater than that at the tympanic membrane for a given driving force simply because of this difference in area. An increase in sound pressure by a factor of 17 corresponds to a decibel increase of 24.6 dB. Thus, of the approximately 30 dB that would be lost if the air-filled outer ear were linked directly to the fluid-filled inner ear, almost 25 dB is recovered due solely to the areal ratio of the eardrum to the stapes footplate.

The other primary mechanism that might contribute to the compensation for the existing impedance mismatch has to do with a complex lever system presumed to exist within the ossicles. The lever is created by the difference in length between the malleus and a portion of the incus known as the long process. This lever factor, however, recovers only approximately 2 dB of the loss due to the impedance mismatch. The assumptions underlying the operation of this lever mechanism, moreover, are not firmly established.

The middle ear system, therefore, compensates for much of the loss of sound energy that would result if the airborne sound waves impinged directly on the fluid-filled inner ear. Approximately 25–27 dB of the estimated 30-dB impedance mismatch has been compensated for by the middle ear. The ability of the middle ear system to amplify or boost the sound pressure is dependent on signal frequency. Specifically, little pressure amplification occurs for frequencies below 100 Hz or above 2000–2500 Hz. Recall, however, that the outer ear amplified sound energy by 20 dB for frequencies from 2000 to 5000 Hz. Thus, taken together, the portion of the auditory system peripheral to the stapes footplate increases sound pressure by 20–25 dB in a range of approximately 100–5000 Hz.

Another, less obvious, function of the middle ear also involves the outer ear/inner ear link formed by the ossicles. Because of the presence of this mechanical link, the preferred pathway for sound vibrations striking the eardrum will be along the chain formed by the three ossicles. Sound energy, therefore, will be routed directly to the oval window. There is another membranous window of the inner ear that also lies along the inner or medial wall of the middle ear cavity. This structure is known as the round window (Fig. 3.1). For the inner ear to be stimulated appropriately by the vibrations of the sound waves, it is important that the oval window and round window not be displaced in the same direction simultaneously. This situation would arise frequently, however, if the sound wave impinged directly upon the medial wall of the middle ear cavity where both the oval window and the round window are located. Thus, routing the vibrations of the eardrum directly to the oval window via the ossicles assures appropriate stimulation of the inner ear.

Finally, we mentioned previously that two tiny muscles are located within the middle ear and make contact with the ossicular chain. These muscles can be made to contract in a variety of situations. Some individuals can contract these muscles voluntarily. For most individuals, however, the contraction is an involuntary reflex arising either from loud acoustic stimuli or from nonacoustic stimuli (such as a puff of air applied to the eyes, or scratching the skin on the face just in front of the external auditory meatus), or accompanying voluntary movements of the oral musculature, as in chewing, swallowing, or yawning. Regarding the reflexive contraction of the middle ear muscles resulting from acoustic stimulation, sound levels must generally exceed 85 dB SPL to elicit a contraction.

The result of middle ear muscle contraction is to stiffen the ossicular chain and to essentially pull the ossicular chain away from the two structures it links, the outer ear and inner ear. This results in an attenuation or decrease of sound pressure reaching the inner ear. The attenuation amounts to 15–20 dB and is frequency dependent. Recall from the previous chapter that increases in a system's stiffness have the greatest effect on low-frequency vibrations. Consequently, the attenuation produced by the middle-ear muscles contracting and increasing the stiffness of the ossicles exists only for frequencies below 2000 Hz. The attenuation measured for acoustically elicited contractions, moreover, appears to apply only to stimuli of high intensities. That is, low-level signals such as those near threshold are not attenuated when middle ear muscle contraction is elicited, but high-level signals (> 80 dB SPL) may be attenuated by as much as 15–20 dB. The middle ear reflex is known as a consensual reflex, meaning that when either ear is appropriately stimulated, the muscles contract in both ears.

Inner Ear

The inner ear is a complex structure that resides deep within a very dense portion of the skull known as the petrous portion of the temporal bone. Because of the complexity of this structure, it is often referred to as a labyrinth. The inner ear consists of a bony outer casing, the osseous labyrinth. Within this bony structure is the membranous labyrinth. The osseous labyrinth, as shown in Figure 3.3, can be divided into three major sections: the *semicircular canals* (*superior, lateral, posterior*); the *vestibule;* and the *cochlea.* The first two sections house the sensory organs for the vestibular system. The vestibular system assists in maintaining balance and posture. The focus here, however, will be placed on the remaining portion of the osseous inner ear, the cochlea. It is the cochlea that contains the sensory organ for hearing. The coiled, snail-shaped cochlea has approximately 2¾ turns in human beings. The largest turn is called the basal turn, while the smallest turn at the top of the cochlea is referred to as the apical turn. Two additional anatomic landmarks of the inner ear depicted in Figure 3.3 are the *oval window* and the *round window.* Recall that the footplate of the stapes is attached to the oval window.

The cochlea is cut in cross section from top to bottom in Figure 3.4. The winding channel running throughout the bony snail-shaped structure is seen to be further subdivided into three compartments. The compartment sandwiched between the other two is a cross section of the membranous labyrinth that runs throughout the osseous labyrinth. All three compartments are filled with fluid. The middle compartment, known as the *scala media,* is filled with a fluid called endolymph. The two adjacent compartments, the *scala vestibuli* and *scala tympani,* contain a different fluid, called perilymph. At the apex of the cochlea is a small hole called the *helicotrema* that connects the two compartments filled with perilymph, the scala tympani and scala vestibuli. The oval window forms an interface

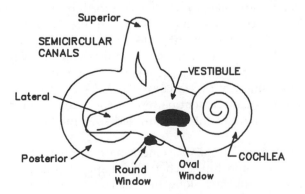

Figure 3.3. Illustration of the osseous labyrinth and its landmarks. (Adapted from Durrant JD, Lovrinic JH: *Bases of Hearing Science,* ed 2. Baltimore, Williams & Wilkins, 1984, p 98.)

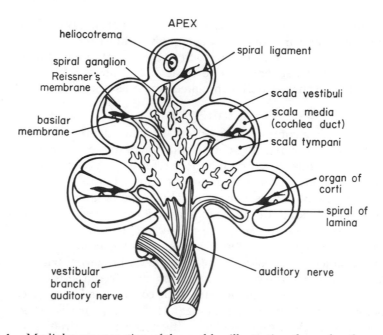

APEX

heliocotrema

spiral ganglion

Reissner's membrane

basilar membrane

spiral ligament

scala vestibuli

scala media (cochlea duct)

scala tympani

organ of corti

spiral of lamina

vestibular branch of auditory nerve

auditory nerve

Figure 3.4.   Modiolar cross section of the cochlea illustrating the scalae through each of the turns. (Adapted from Zemlin WR: *Speech and Hearing Science: Anatomy and Physiology,* ed 2. Englewood Cliffs, NJ, Prentice-Hall, 1988, p 464.)

between the ossicular chain of the middle ear and the fluid-filled scala vestibuli of the inner ear. When the oval window vibrates as a consequence of vibration of the ossicular chain, a wave is established within the scala vestibuli. Because the fluid-filled compartments are essentially sealed within the osseous labyrinth, the inward displacement of the cochlear fluids at the oval window must be matched by an outward displacement elsewhere. This is accomplished via the round window, which communicates directly with the scala tympani. When the oval window is pushed inward by the stapes, the round window is pushed outward by the increased pressure in the inner ear fluid.

When the stapes footplate rocks back and forth in the oval window, a wave is created within the cochlear fluids. This wave displaces the scala media in a wavelike manner. This displacement pattern is usually simplified by considering the motion of just one of the partitions forming the scala media, the *basilar membrane*. The motion depicted for the basilar membrane, however, also occurs for the opposite partition of the scala media, *Reissner's membrane*. Although we will be depicting the displacement pattern of the basilar membrane, the reader should bear in mind that the entire fluid-filled scala media is undergoing similar displacement.

Figure 3.5 illustrates the displacement pattern of the basilar membrane at four successive instants in time. When this displacement pattern is visualized directly, the wave established along the basilar membrane is seen to move or travel from the base to the apex. The displacement pattern increases gradually in amplitude as it progresses from the base toward the apex until it reaches a point of maximum displacement. At that point, the amplitude of displacement

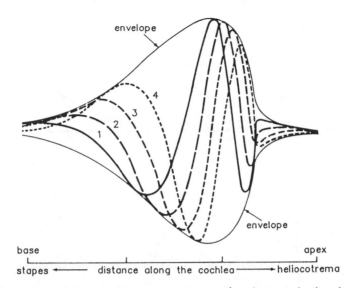

Figure 3.5. Illustration of the traveling wave pattern at four instants in time in response to a mid-frequency sound. The *thin solid lines* connect the maximum and minimum displacements at each location along the cochlea and for each instant in time. These *thin solid lines* represent the envelope of the displacement patterns. (Adapted from von Bekesy G: *Experiments in Hearing.* New York, McGraw-Hill, 1960, p 462.)

decreases abruptly. The *thin solid line* connecting the amplitude peaks at various locations for these four instants in time describes the displacement envelope. The envelope pattern is symmetrical in that the same pattern superimposed on the positive peaks can be flipped upside down and used to describe the negative peaks. As a result, only the positive or upper half of the envelope describing maximum displacement is usually displayed.

Figure 3.6 displays the envelopes of the displacement pattern of the basilar membrane that have been observed for different stimulus frequencies. Note that, as the frequency of the stimulus increases, the peak of the displacement pattern moves in a basal direction closer to the stapes footplate. At low frequencies, virtually the entire membrane undergoes some degree of displacement. As stimulus frequency increases, a more restricted region of the basilar membrane undergoes displacement. Thus, the cochlea is performing a crude frequency analysis of the incoming sound. In general, for all but the very low frequencies (< 50 Hz), there is a correspondence between the place of maximum displacement within the cochlea and the frequency of the stimulus. The frequency of the acoustic stimulus striking the eardrum and displacing the stapes footplate will be analyzed or distinguished from sounds of different frequency by the location of the displacement pattern along the basilar membrane.

Because the pressure wave created within the cochlear fluids originates near the base of the cochlea at the oval window, one might think that this is the reason the traveling wave displacement pattern appears to move from the base to the apex. On the contrary, experiments with models of the inner ear have shown that the source of vibration (oval window) can be located anywhere along the cochlea, including the apex, with no effect on the displacement pattern of the

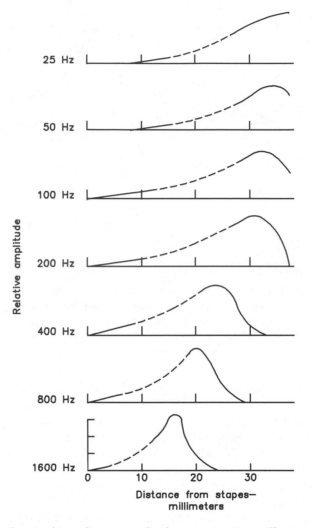

Figure 3.6. Envelopes of traveling wave displacement patterns illustrated for different stimulus frequencies. Notice that low frequencies (*top*) produce a maximum displacement of the basilar membrane in the apex (farthest distance from the stapes), while higher frequencies (*bottom*) produce maximum displacement in the basal portion of the cochlea (nearer to the stapes). (Adapted from von Bekesy G: *Experiments in Hearing*. New York, McGraw-Hill, 1960, p 448).

basilar membrane (Vignette 3.1). The primary physical feature of the inner ear responsible for the direction in which the traveling wave progresses is the stiffness gradient of the basilar membrane. The stiffness of the basilar membrane decreases from the base to the apex.

A more detailed picture of the structures within the scala media is provided in Figure 3.7. The sensory organ of hearing, the organ of Corti, is seen to rest on top of the basilar membrane (BM). The organ of Corti contains several thousand sensory receptor cells called *hair cells*. Each hair cell has several tiny hairs or cilia protruding from the top of the cell. As shown in Figure 3.7, there are two types

---

Vignette 3.1. Discussion of the Traveling-Wave Paradox

As mentioned, regardless of where the vibration is introduced into the cochlea, the traveling wave always travels from base to apex. This phenomenon is known as the traveling wave paradox. The early tests of hearing that were routinely performed decades ago with tuning forks made use of this phenomenon. A tuning fork was struck, and the vibrating tongs were placed next to the outer ear. The tester asked the listener to indicate when the tone produced by the vibrating tuning fork could no longer be heard. Immediately after the listener indicated that the sound was no longer audible, the base of the tuning fork was pressed against the bony portion of the skull known as the mastoid process, immediately behind the ear. If the listener could now hear the tone again, it was assumed that the hearing sensitivity of the inner ear alone was better than that of the entire peripheral portion of the auditory system as a whole (outer ear, middle ear, and inner ear).

When the base of the tuning fork was placed on the mastoid process, the skull was vibrated. The cochlea is imbedded firmly within the temporal bone of the skull, such that skull vibrations produce a mechanical vibration of the inner ear. Even though the vibration is not introduced at the oval window by the vibrating stapes, the tone produced by the tuning fork placed against the skull is still heard as though it were. The traveling wave within the inner ear behaves the same, regardless of where the mechanical vibration is introduced.

For normal listeners, the typical means of stimulating the inner ear is through the outer and middle ears. This is known as air conduction hearing. Sound can also be introduced by vibrating the skull at the mastoid process, forehead, or some other location. This is called bone conduction hearing. Whether the tone is introduced into the inner ear by bone conduction or air conduction, the traveling wave and the resulting sensation are the same.

Modern-day air conduction and bone conduction tests are described in more detail in Chapter 4. They are of great assistance in determining which portion of the peripheral auditory system is impaired in listeners with hearing loss.

---

of hair cells within the organ of Corti. The inner hair cells (IHC) comprise a single row of receptors located closest to the modiolus or bony core of the cochlea. The cilia of these cells are free standing, i.e., they do not make contact with any other structures. Approximately 90–95% of the auditory nerve fibers (NF) that carry information to the brain make contact with the inner hair cells. The outer hair cells (OHC) are much greater in number and are usually organized in three rows. The cilia of the outer hair cells are embedded within a gelatinous structure known as the *tectorial membrane* (TM), draped over the top of the organ of Corti.

Note that the organ of Corti is bordered by two membranes: the basilar membrane below and the tectorial membrane above. The modiolar or medial points of attachment for these two membranes are offset. That is, the tectorial membrane is attached to a structure called the spiral limbus, which is located nearer to the modiolus than the comparable point of attachment for the basilar membrane (a bony structure called the spiral lamina). Figure 3.8 illustrates one of the consequences of these staggered points of attachment. When the basilar membrane is displaced in an upward direction (toward the scala vestibuli), the cilia of the outer hair cells embedded in the tectorial membrane undergo a

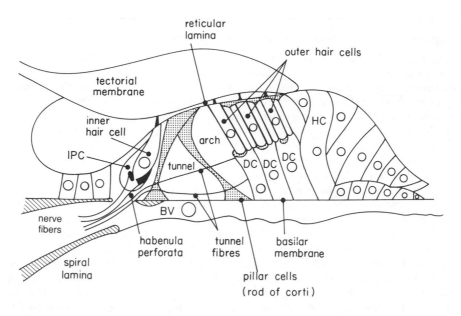

Figure 3.7. Detailed cross section of the organ of Corti. *IPC,* inner pillar cell; *BV,* basilar vessel; *DC,* Deiter cell; and *HC,* Hensen cell. (Adapted from Pickles JO: *An Introduction to the Physiology of Hearing,* ed 2. London, Academic Press, 1988, p 29).

shearing force in a radial direction (a horizontal direction in the figure). Displacement in a downward direction develops a radial shearing force in the opposite direction. This shearing force is believed to be the trigger that initiates a series of electrical and chemical processes within the hair cells. This, in turn, leads to the activation of the auditory nerve fibers that are in contact with the base of the hair cell.

The two primary functions of the auditory portion of the inner ear can be summarized as follows. First, the inner ear performs a frequency analysis on incoming sounds so that different frequencies stimulate different regions of the inner ear. Second, mechanical vibration is converted into electrical energy by the hair cells.

Auditory Nerve

The action potentials generated by auditory nerve fibers are called all-or-none potentials. That is, they do not vary in amplitude when activated. If the nerve fibers fire, they always fire to the same degree, reaching 100% amplitude. The action potentials, moreover, are very short-lived events, typically requiring less than 1–2 ms to rise in amplitude to maximum potential and return to resting state. For this reason, they are frequently referred to as spikes. They can be recorded by inserting a tiny microelectrode into a nerve fiber. When this is done, spikes can be observed even without the presentation of an acoustic stimulus. That is, the nerve fiber has spontaneous activity that consists of random firings of the nerve fiber. The lowest sound intensity that gives rise to a criterion percentage increase (e.g., 20% increase) in the rate at which the fiber is firing is called the threshold for that particular stimulus frequency. As stimulus intensity

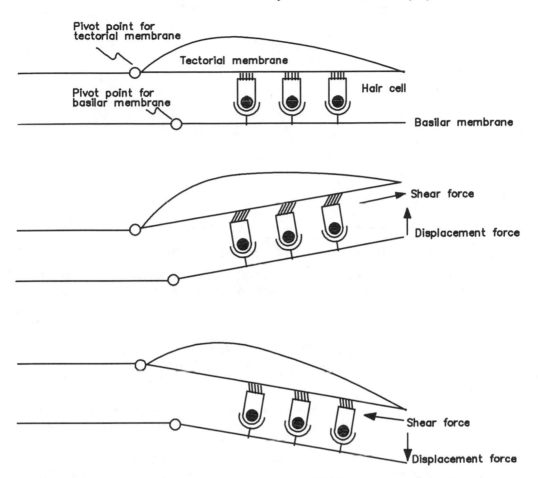

Figure 3.8. Illustration of the mechanism responsible for the generation of shearing forces on the cilia of the outer hair cells. Because the pivot points for the tectorial membrane and basilar membrane, represented in each drawing by the *small circles,* are offset horizontally, displacement of the basilar membrane in a vertical direction creates shearing forces across the cilia in a radial direction (i.e., a push or pull of the cilia in a horizontal left-to-right direction in the drawings) (Adapted from Zemlin WR: *Speech and Hearing Science: Anatomy and Physiology,* ed 2. Englewood Cliffs, NJ, Prentice-Hall, p 484).

is raised above threshold, the amplitude of the spikes does not change. They always fire at maximum response. The rate at which the nerve fiber responds, however, does increase with stimulus level. This is illustrated in Figure 3.9, in which an input-output function for a single auditory nerve fiber is displayed. Note that the discharge rate, or *spike rate,* increases steadily with input level above the spontaneous rate until a maximum discharge rate is reached approximately 30–40 dB above threshold. Consequently, a single nerve fiber can code intensity via the discharge rate over only a limited range of intensities. Again, an increase in intensity is encoded by an increase in the firing rate (more spikes per second), not by an increase in the amplitude of the response.

The *solid line* in Figure 3.10c depicts the frequency-threshold curve (FTC) of a single auditory nerve fiber. Combinations of stimulus intensity and frequency

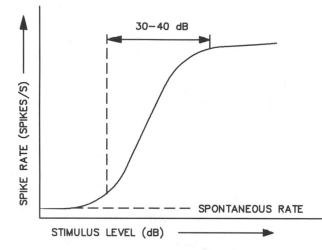

Figure 3.9. An input-output function for a single auditory nerve fiber. As stimulus intensity increases, the firing rate of the nerve fiber increases, but only over a narrow range of 30–40 dB.

lying within the *hatched area* bordered by the FTC will cause the nerve fiber to increase its firing rate above the spontaneous rate. Frequency/intensity combinations lying outside this region fail to activate the nerve fiber. The *hatched region*, therefore, is frequently referred to as the nerve fiber's response area.

Note that the FTC for the nerve fiber in Figure 3.10c indicates that the nerve fiber responds best to a frequency of 2000 Hz. That is, 2000 Hz is the frequency requiring the least amount of stimulus intensity to evoke a response from the nerve fiber. This frequency is referred to often as the best frequency or characteristic frequency of the nerve fiber. There are some nerve fibers that have a low characteristic frequency and some that have a high characteristic frequency. This is illustrated in the other panels of Figure 3.10. Those fibers having high characteristic frequencies come from hair cells in the base, while those having low characteristic frequencies supply the apex. As the nerve fibers exit through the bony core of the cochlea, or modiolus, on their way to the brainstem, they maintain an orderly arrangement. The bundle of nerve fibers comprising the cochlear branch of the auditory nerve is organized so that fibers having high characteristic frequencies are located around the perimeter, while fibers having low characteristic frequencies comprise the core of the cochlear nerve. Thus, the auditory nerve is organized, as is the basilar membrane, so that each characteristic frequency corresponds to a place within the nerve bundle. This mapping of frequency of the sound wave to place of maximum activity within an anatomic structure is referred to as tonotopic organization.

Temporal or time-domain information is also coded by fibers of the auditory nerve. Consider, for example, the discharge pattern that occurs within a nerve fiber when that stimulus is a sinusoid that lies within the response area of the nerve fiber. The pattern of spikes that occurs under such conditions is illustrated in Figure 3.11a. Note that when the single nerve fiber discharges, it always does so at essentially the same location on the stimulus waveform. In Figure 3.11a this

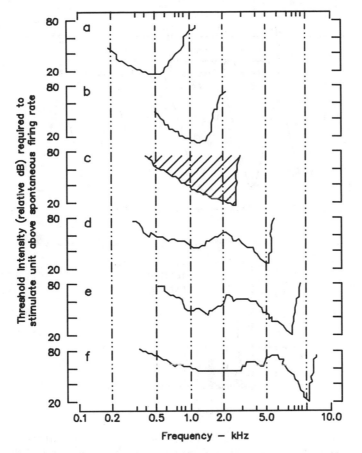

Figure 3.10. Frequency-threshold curves (FTCs) for 6 auditory nerve fibers (*a–f*). The FTC illustrates the intensity required at each frequency to just produce a measurable response in the nerve fiber. The frequency requiring the lowest intensity for a response is known as the "best frequency" or "characteristic frequency." The best frequency for each of the six nerve fibers increases from top (*a*) to bottom (*f*). The area within each curve, illustrated in *c* by the *hatched region*, represents the response area of the nerve fiber. Any combination of frequency and intensity represented in that area will yield a response from the nerve fiber.

happens to be the positive peak of the waveform. Notice also that it may not fire during every cycle of the stimulus waveform. Nonetheless, if one were to record the time interval between successive spikes and examine the number of times each interval occurred, a histogram of the results would look like that shown in Figure 3.11**b**. This histogram, known simply as an interval histogram, indicates that the most frequent interspike interval corresponds to the period of the waveform. All other peaks in the histogram occur at integer multiples of the period. Thus, the nerve fiber is able to encode the period of the waveform. This holds true for nerve fibers having characteristic frequencies less than approximately 2000 Hz. As discussed in Chapter 2, if we know the period of a sinusoidal waveform, we know its frequency ($f=1/T$). Hence, the nerve fibers responding in the manner depicted in Figure 3.11 could code the frequency of the acoustic

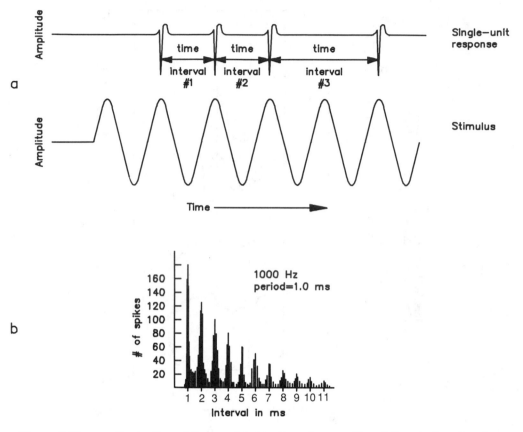

Figure 3.11. **a,** Illustration of the synchronization of nerve fiber firings to the stimulus waveform. Note that the nerve fiber always fires at the same point of the waveform, although it may not fire every cycle. The time intervals between successive firings of the nerve fiber can be measured and stored for later analysis. **b,** A histogram of the intervals measured in **a,** referred to as interspike intervals. An interval of 1 ms was the most frequently occurring interval, having occurred about 180 times. This corresponds to the period of the waveform in **a.**

stimulus according to the timing of discharges. For frequencies up to 5000 Hz, the neural firing is synchronized to the sound stimulus as in the upper portion of Figure 3.11. By combining synchronized firings for several nerve fibers, it is possible to encode the period of sounds up to 5000 Hz in frequency.

The electrical activity of the auditory nerve can also be recorded from more remote locations. In this case, however, the action potentials are not being measured from single nerve fibers. Recorded electrical activity under these circumstances represents the composite response from a large number of nerve fibers. For this reason, this composite electrical response is referred to frequently as the whole-nerve action potential. The whole-nerve action potential can be recorded in human subjects from the ear canal or from the medial wall of the middle ear cavity by placing a needle electrode through the eardrum. Because the whole-nerve action potential represents the summed activity of several nerve fibers, the more fibers can be made to fire simultaneously, the greater the amplitude of the response. For this reason, brief abrupt acoustic signals, such as clicks or short-duration pure tones, are used as stimuli. Recall, however, that the traveling wave begins in the base and travels toward the apex. It takes roughly 2–4 ms for the traveling wave to travel the full length of the cochlea from the base to apex. Even for abrupt stimuli, such as clicks, the nerve fibers are not triggered simultaneously throughout the cochlea. Fibers associated with the basal high-frequency region respond synchronously to the stimulus presentation. Those fibers originating further up the cochlea will fire later (up to 2–4 ms later). Those firing in synchrony will provide the largest contribution to the whole-nerve action potential. Consequently, the whole-nerve action potential does not represent the activity of the entire nerve but reflects primarily the response of the synchronous high-frequency fibers associated with the base of the cochlea.

The input-output function for the whole-nerve action potential differs considerably from that described previously for single nerve fibers. For the whole-nerve action potential, the response is measured in terms of its amplitude or latency, not spike rate. The input-output function of the whole-nerve action potential shows a steady increase in amplitude with increase in stimulus level. This is illustrated in Figure 3.12. Also shown is a plot of the latency of the response as a function of stimulus intensity. Latency refers to the time intervening between stimulus onset and the onset of the neural response. Note that, as stimulus intensity is increased, the latency of the response decreases. Thus, as response amplitude increases with intensity, response latency decreases. The plot of re-

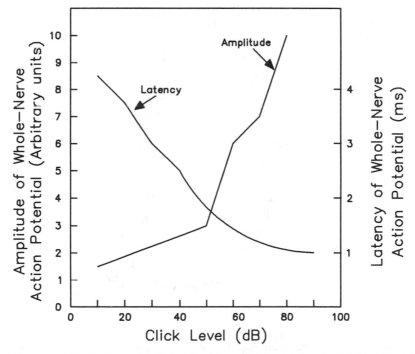

Figure 3.12.   Amplitude-intensity (*left ordinate*) and latency-intensity (*right ordinate*) functions for the whole-nerve action potential. As intensity increases, the *amplitude* of the action potential increases and the latency of the response decreases.

sponse latency as a function of stimulus intensity is called a latency-intensity function. The latency-intensity function is of primary importance in clinical electrophysiologic assessment of auditory function.

AUDITORY CENTRAL NERVOUS SYSTEM

Once the action potentials have been generated in the cochlear branch of the auditory nerve, the electrical activity progresses up toward the cortex. This network of nerve fibers is frequently referred to as the auditory central nervous system (auditory CNS). The nerve fibers that carry information in the form of action potentials up the auditory CNS toward the cortex form part of the ascending or afferent pathways. Nerve impulses can also be sent toward the periphery from the cortex or brainstem centers. The fibers carrying such information comprise the descending or efferent pathways.

Figure 3.13 provides a simplified schematic diagram of the ascending auditory CNS. All nerve fibers from the cochlea terminate at the cochlear nucleus on the same side. From here, however, several possible paths are available. The majority of nerve fibers cross over or decussate at some point along the auditory CNS, so that the activity of the right ear is represented most strongly on the left side of the cortex and vice versa. The crossover, however, is not complete. From the superior olives through the cortex, activity from both ears is represented on

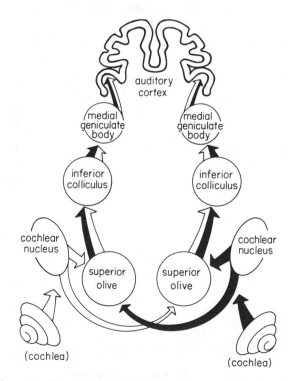

Figure 3.13. Schematic illustration of the ascending pathways of the central auditory nervous system. The *black arrows* represent input from the right ear, while the *white arrows* represent input from the left ear. (Adapted from Yost WA, Nielsen DW: *Fundamentals of Hearing: An Introduction*, ed 2. New York, Holt, Rinehart, & Winston, 1985, p 98.)

each side. All ascending fibers terminate in the medial geniculate body before ascending to the cortex. Thus, all ascending fibers within the brainstem portion of the auditory CNS synapse at the cochlear nucleus and at the medial geniculate body, taking one of several paths between these two points, with many paths having additional intervening nerve fibers. Vignette 3.2 describes measurement of the auditory brainstem response and its correlation with anatomic structure.

We have reviewed previously the simple coding of information available in the responses of the auditory nerve fibers. The mapping of frequency to place within the cochlea, for example, was seen to be preserved in the responses of the nerve fibers in that fibers having high characteristic frequencies originated from the high-frequency base of the cochlea. The period of the waveform could also be coded for stimulus frequencies less than 5000 Iz. In addition, the intensity of the stimulus was coded over a limited range (30–40 dB) by the discharge rate of the fiber. At the level of the cochlear nucleus, it is already apparent that the ascending auditory pathway begins processing information by converting this fairly simple code into more complex codes. The coding of timing information is much more complex. In addition, some nerve fibers within the cochlear nucleus have a much broader range of intensities (up to 100 dB) over which the discharge rate increases steadily with sound intensity. As one probes nerve fibers at various centers within the auditory CNS, a tremendous diversity of responses is evident.

Despite this increasing anatomic and physiologic complexity, one thing that appears to be preserved throughout the auditory CNS is tonotopic organization. At each brainstem center and within the auditory portions of the cortex, there is an orderly mapping of frequency to place. This can be demonstrated by measuring the characteristic frequency of nerve fibers encountered at various locations within a given brainstem center or within the cortex.

Another principle underlying the auditory CNS is that of redundancy. That is, information represented in the neural code from one ear has multiple representations at various locations within the auditory system. Every auditory nerve fiber, for example, splits into two fibers before entering the cochlear nucleus, with each branch supplying a different region of the cochlear nucleus. In addition, from the superior olives through the auditory areas of the cortex, information from both ears is represented.

Our knowledge of the ascending pathway of the auditory CNS is far from complete. We know even less, however, about the descending pathways. This is due, in part, to the small number of efferent nerve fibers involved in this pathway. There are about two descending efferent fibers for every 100 ascending afferent nerve fibers. Essentially the same brainstem centers are involved in the descending pathway as were involved in the ascending path, although an entirely separate set of nerve fibers is used. The last fiber in this descending pathway runs from the superior olivary complex to enter the cochlea on the same side or the cochlea on the opposite side. These fibers are referred to as either the crossed or uncrossed olivocochlear bundles. The vast majority (60–80%) of these fibers cross over from the superior olivary complex on one side to the cochlea on the other side and innervate the outer hair cells. The remaining fibers comprise the uncrossed bundle and appear to innervate the inner hair cells.

All descending fibers do not terminate at the cochlear nerve fibers. Decending fibers may modify incoming neurally coded sensory information at any of

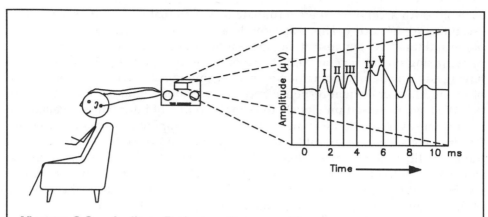

Vignette 3.2.   Auditory Brainstem Response Measurements

It was mentioned earlier that the whole-nerve action potential represented the summed response of many single nerve fibers firing synchronously in response to an abrupt acoustic signal. It was also mentioned that this potential can be recorded remotely from the ear canal. The left-hand portion of the drawing that accompanies this vignette shows a schematic drawing of a patient with electrodes pasted to the skin of the forehead, the top of the head (vertex), and the mastoid. The tracing in the right-hand portion of this illustration shows the electrical activity recorded from the patient. The acoustic stimulus is a brief click that produces synchronized responses from nerve fibers in the cochlea and the brainstem portion of the auditory CNS. The tracing represents the average of 2000 stimulus presentations presented at a moderate intensity at a rate of 11 clicks per second. Approximately 3 minutes is required to present all 2000 stimuli and to obtain the average response shown above. Note that the time scale for the x axis of the tracing spans from 0 to 10 ms. This represents a 10-ms interval beginning with the onset of the click stimulus. The tracing shows several distinct bumps or waves, with the first appearing at about 1.5 ms after stimulus onset. This first wave, labeled *I*, is believed to be a remote recording of the whole-nerve action potential from the closest portion of the auditory nerve. Approximately 1 ms later, 2.5 ms after stimulus onset, wave *II* is observed. This wave is believed to be the response of the more distant portion of the auditory nerve. One millisecond later the electrical activity has travelled to the next center in the brainstem, the cochlear nucleus, and produces the response recorded as wave *III*. Wave *IV* represents the activity of the superior olivary complex. Wave *V* represents the response of the lateral lemniscus, a structure lying between the superior olives and the inferior colliculus. Waves *VI* and *VII* (the two unlabeled bumps after Wave *V*) represent the response of the latter brainstem structure.

The response shown in the right-hand tracing is known as an auditory brainstem response (ABR). It has proven very useful in a wide variety of clinical applications, from assessment of the functional integrity of the peripheral and brainstem portions of the ascending auditory CNS to assessment of hearing in infants or difficult-to-test patients.

the centers along the auditory CNS. In addition, they may either facilitate or inhibit responses along the ascending auditory pathway. That is, electrical stimulation of some descending fibers increases the discharges recorded from fibers at lower centers, while stimulation of other descending fibers results in decreased activity at lower centers. Thus, the descending efferent system regulates, modifies, and shapes the incoming sensory information.

Reflexive contractions of the middle ear muscles due to the presentation of a sound stimulus may also be considered as a regulating mechanism for the incoming sensory information. The reflex pathway is illustrated schematically in Figure 3.14. Incoming sensory information enters through the peripheral auditory system and ascends to the superior olive. If the sound is sufficiently intense, descending information is routed to motor nuclei that control the contraction of the middle ear muscles. This explains why the reflexive contraction of middle ear muscles due to sound stimuli is a consensual phenomenon, as mentioned previously. Information from the cochlear nucleus goes to both superior olives, so that sound stimulation on one side yields middle ear muscle contraction on both sides.

PERCEPTION OF SOUND

Having reviewed the basic structure and some key aspects of the physiologic function of the auditory system, the remainder of this chapter reviews some fundamental aspects of the perception of sound by humans. We have examined the acoustics involved in the generation and propagation of a sound wave and have reviewed its conversion into a complex neural code. This code of incoming sensory information can influence the behavior of a human subject, whether the sound is the loud whistle of an oncoming train or the cry of a hungry infant. The study of behavioral responses to acoustic stimulation is referred to as psychoacoustics.

Psychoacoustics

Psychoacoustics is the study of the relationship between the sound stimulus and the behavioral response it produces in the subject. We have already discussed how the important parameters of the acoustic stimulus can be measured. Much of psychoacoustics concerns itself with the more challenging task of appropriately measuring the listener's response. Two primary means have evolved through

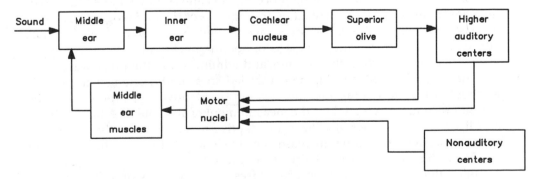

Figure 3.14.   Schematic illustration of the reflex arc for the middle ear muscle reflex.

which the psychoacoustician measures responses from the listener. The first, known generally as the discrimination procedure, is used to assess the smallest difference that would allow a listener to discriminate between two stimulus conditions. The end result is an estimate of a threshold of a certain type. A tone of specified amplitude, frequency, and starting phase, for example, can be discriminated from the absence of such a signal. In this particular case, one is measuring the absolute threshold for hearing. That is, the absolute threshold is a statistical concept that represents the lowest sound pressure level at which the tone can be heard a certain percentage of the time. This threshold is often referred to as a detection threshold, because one is determining the stimulus parameters required to just detect the presence of a signal.

Discrimination procedures have also been used to measure difference thresholds. A difference threshold is a statistical concept that indicates the smallest change in a stimulus that can be just detected by the listener. A standard sound that is fixed in intensity, frequency, starting phase, and duration is employed. A comparison stimulus that differs typically in one of these stimulus parameters is then presented. The difference threshold indicates how much the comparison stimulus must differ from the standard signal to permit detection of the difference by the listener a certain percentage of the time.

Many of the discrimination procedures used to measure absolute and difference thresholds were developed over a century ago. Three such procedures, referred to as the classic psychophysical methods, are: (a) the method of limits; (b) the method of adjustment; and (c) the method of constant stimuli. Research conducted in more recent years has resulted in two important developments regarding the use of these procedures. First, it was recognized that thresholds measured with these procedures were not uncontaminated estimates of sensory function. Rather, thresholds measured with these procedures could be altered considerably by biasing the subject through various means, such as the use of different sets of instructions or different schedules of reinforcement for correct and incorrect responses. The threshold for the detection of a low-intensity pure tone, for example, can be changed by instructing the listener to be very certain that a tone was heard before responding accordingly, or by encouraging the listener to guess when uncertain. The magnitude of sensation evoked within the sensory system during stimulus presentation should remain unchanged under these manipulations. Yet the threshold was noticeably affected. Threshold as measured with any of these classic procedures is affected by factors other than the magnitude of sensation evoked by the signal. For the audiologist, however, the classic psychophysical procedures have proven to be valid and reliable tools with which to measure various aspects of hearing in clinical settings as long as care is used in instructing the listeners and administering the procedures.

The second recent development that led to a modification of the classic psychophysical procedures was the creation of adaptive test procedures. The current procedure advocated for the measurement of absolute threshold of hearing (discussed in Chapter 4) utilizes an adaptive modification of the method of limits. Adaptive procedures increase the efficiency of the paradigm without sacrificing the accuracy or reliability of the procedure.

In addition to discrimination procedures, a second class of techniques has been developed to quantify subjects' responses to acoustic signals. These procedures, known generally as scaling techniques, attempt to measure sensation directly. In the study of hearing, they are used most frequently to measure the sensation of loudness, though they have also been used to quantify other sensations, such as pitch. The results from one of these procedures, magnitude estimation, are shown in Figure 3.15. In the magnitude estimation technique, subjects simply assign numbers to the perceived loudness of a series of stimuli. In the case shown in Figure 3.15, the stimuli differed only in intensity. The average results fall along a straight line when plotted on log-log coordinates. Both the x axis and y axis in Figure 3.15 are logarithmic. Recall that the decibel scale, the x axis in this figure, involved the logarithm of a pressure ratio, i.e., SPL in dB = 20 log (p_1/p_2). Comparable results have been obtained for other sensations, such as brightness, vibration on the fingertip, and electric shock. In all cases, a straight line fits the average data very well when plotted on log-log coordinates. From these extensive data, a law was developed which relates the perceived magnitude of sensation (S) to the physical intensity of the stimulus (I) in the following manner: $S=kI^x$, where k is an arbitrary constant and x is an exponent that varies with the sensation under investigation. This law is known as Stevens' power law in honor of the scientist S. S. Stevens, who discovered and developed it. A convenient feature of a power function plotted on log-log coordinates is that the slope of the line fit to the data is the exponent, x.

Finally, a procedure that has been used extensively in psychoacoustics to measure auditory sensations via the subject's response is the matching procedure. The matching procedure is a cross between discrimination procedures and scaling procedures in that the technique is similar to that of the method of adjustment (one of the classic psychophysical methods) but its goal is to quantify a subjective attribute of sound, such as loudness or pitch. The matching proce-

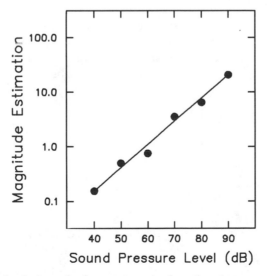

Figure 3.15. Hypothetical results from a magnitude estimation experiment in which the perceived loudness was measured for various sound levels. Note that the results fall along a straight line when both axes are logarithmic (recall that the dB scale incorporates logarithms in the calculation of dB).

dures enable the experimenter to determine a set of stimulus parameters that all yield the same subjective sensation. A pure tone fixed at 1000 Hz and 70 dB SPL, for example, may be presented to one ear of a listener and a second pure tone of 8000 Hz presented to the other ear in an alternating fashion. The subject controls the intensity of the 8000-Hz tone until it is judged to be equal in loudness to the 1000-Hz, 70-dB SPL reference tone. Data in the literature indicate that the 8000-Hz tone would have to be set to 80–85 dB SPL to achieve a loudness match in the case presented above.

Hearing Threshold

Let us now examine how these procedures have been applied to the study of the perception of sound. The results obtained from the measurement of hearing thresholds at various frequencies are depicted in Figure 3.16. Note that the sound pressure level that is just detectable varies with frequency, especially below 500 Hz and above 8000 Hz. The slope of the function in the low frequencies is due to the attenuation of lower frequencies by the middle ear. It is apparent that the contour of the hearing threshold has a minimum in the 2000- to 4000-Hz range. This is attributable, in large part, to the amplification of signals in this frequency range by the outer ear, as discussed earlier in this chapter. The range of audibility of the normal-hearing human ear is described frequently as 20–20,000 Hz. That is, frequencies above or below this range typically cannot be heard by the normal human ear.

Masking

The phenomenon of masking has also been studied in detail. Masking refers to the ability of one acoustic signal to obscure the presence of another acoustic signal so that it cannot be detected. A whisper might be audible, for example, in a quiet environment. In a noisy industrial environment, however, such a weak acoustic signal would be masked by the more intense factory noise.

The masking of pure tone signals by noise has been studied extensively. To consider the results that have been obtained, however, we must first examine some important acoustic characteristics of the masking noise. Briefly, there are two measures of intensity that can be used to describe the level of a noise. These

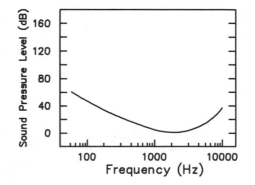

Figure 3.16. Average normal threshold sound pressure level plotted as a function of frequency for binaural (two-ear) listening in a free field (Adapted from Sivian LJ, White SD: Minimum audible pressure and minimum audible field. *J Acoust Soc Am* 4:288–321, 1933.)

two measures are the total power (*TP*) and the noise power per unit (1-Hz) bandwidth, or spectral density (N_o). The total power in dB SPL is the quantity measured by most measuring devices, such as sound level meters. The spectral density of the noise, on the other hand, is not measured directly. Rather, it is calculated from the following equation: $10 \log_{10} N_o = 10 \log_{10} TP - 10 \log_{10} BW$, where *BW* is the bandwidth of the noise in Hz. The quantity $10 \log_{10} N_o$ is the spectrum level in units of dB SPL/Hz and represents the average noise power in a 1-Hz band. For broad-band noises, the spectrum level determines the masking produced at various frequencies.

Figure 3.17 illustrates data obtained from one of the early studies of masking produced by broad-band noise. These data have been replicated several times since. The lowest curve in this figure depicts the threshold in a quiet environment, while all other curves represent masked thresholds obtained for various levels of the noise masker. These levels are expressed as the spectrum level of the masker. Note that the lowest noise levels are not effective maskers at low frequencies. That is, thresholds measured for low-frequency pure tones in the presence of a broad-band noise having $N_o=0$ dB SPL/Hz are the same as in quiet. At all frequencies, however, once the noise begins to produce some masking, a 10-dB increase in noise intensity produces a 10-dB increase in masked threshold for the pure tone. Once the noise level that just begins to produce masking is determined, the desired amount of masking can be produced by simply increasing the noise level by a corresponding amount.

How might the masking produced by a noise be affected by decreasing the bandwidth of the noise? Figure 3.18 illustrates data obtained several decades ago from a now classic masking experiment. The results of this experiment, referred to frequently as the "band-narrowing" experiment, have also been replicated several times since. Masked threshold in dB SPL is plotted as a function of the bandwidth of the masker in Hz. Results for two different pure-tone frequencies are shown. The *unfilled circles* represent data for a 1000-Hz pure tone, and the *filled circles* depict data for a 4000-Hz pure tone. When the band of masking noise

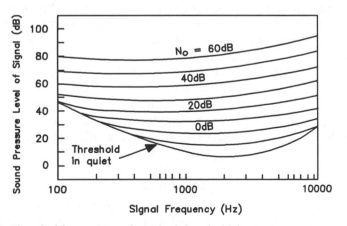

Figure 3.17. Threshold in quiet and masked threshold for various noise spectrum levels (N_o). Threshold was measured at several frequencies in the presence of a broad-band noise. (Adapted from Hawkins JE Jr, Stevens SS: The masking of pure tones and of speech by white noise. *J Acoust Soc Am* 22:6–13, 1950.)

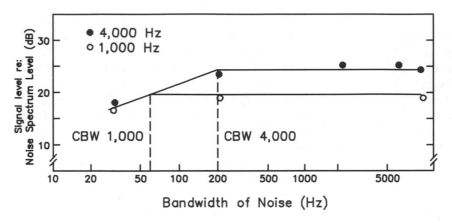

Figure 3.18. Results from the band-narrowing experiment of Fletcher H: Auditory patterns. *Rev Mod Phys* 12:47–65, 1940. Data for two frequencies, 1000 and 4000 Hz, are shown. The critical bandwidths at each frequency are illustrated by *dashed vertical lines*. Note that for bandwidths greater than the critical bandwidth (*CBW*), masking remained unchanged.

was narrowed, the tone was kept in the center of the noise, and the spectrum level of the noise was held constant. For both frequencies, the masked threshold remains the same as the bandwidth decreases, down to a bandwidth called the critical bandwidth. Continued decreases in bandwidth beyond the critical bandwidth reduce the masking produced by the noise, as reflected in the decrease in masked threshold.

The critical bandwidth, first derived from the band-narrowing masking experiment, has proven to be a concept that applies to a wide variety of psychoacoustic phenomena. For the audiologist, however, one of the most important implications drawn from the band-narrowing experiment just described is that a band of noise having a bandwidth just exceeding the critical bandwidth is as effective a masker for a pure tone centered in the noise as a broad-band noise of the same spectrum level. As we will see in the next chapter, the audiologist frequently needs to introduce masking into a patient's ear. A broad-band masking noise can be uncomfortably loud to a patient. The loudness of the noise, however, can be reduced by decreasing the bandwidth of the noise while maintaining the same spectrum level. A masking noise having a bandwidth only slightly greater than the critical bandwidth will be just as effective as broad-band noise in terms of its masking, but much less loud. The narrower-band noise would be more appropriate for use as a masking sound with patients because of its reduced loudness but equal masking capability.

Loudness

Loudness is another psychoacoustic phenomenon that has been studied extensively. The effects of signal bandwidth on loudness, alluded to in the discussion of masking, for instance, have been investigated in detail. Basically, as the bandwidth of the stimulus increases beyond the critical bandwidth, an increasing number of adjacent critical bands are stimulated, resulting in an increase in loudness. Thus, broad-band signals are louder than narrow-band signals at the same spectrum level.

For pure tones, loudness also varies with frequency. This has been established using the matching procedure described previously. Figure 3.19 depicts so-called equal-loudness contours that have been derived with this technique. A given contour displays the sound pressure levels at various frequencies that are required so as to match the loudness of a 1000-Hz pure tone at the level indicated by the contour. For example, note that on the curve labeled *20*, the function coincides with a sound pressure level of 20 dB SPL at 1000 Hz, while on the curve labeled *60*, the function corresponds to 60 dB SPL at 1000 Hz. The contour labeled *60* indicates those combinations of frequencies and intensities that were matched in loudness to a 60-dB SPL, 1000-Hz pure tone. All combinations of stimulus intensity and frequency lying along that contour are said to have a loudness level of 60 phons (correctly pronounced "phones" as in "telephones"). Thus, a 125-Hz pure tone at 70 dB SPL (point labeled *A* in Fig. 3.19) and an 8000-Hz tone at 58 dB SPL (point labeled *B*) are equivalent in loudness to a 60-dB SPL, 1000-Hz pure tone. All three of those stimuli have a loudness level of 60 phons.

Notice in Figure 3.19 that stimulus intensity must be increased by 110 dB in order to go from a loudness level of 10 phons (threshold) to 120 phons at 1000 Hz. At 100 Hz, only an 80-dB increase is required to span that same change in loudness. From this we can conclude that loudness increases more rapidly at low

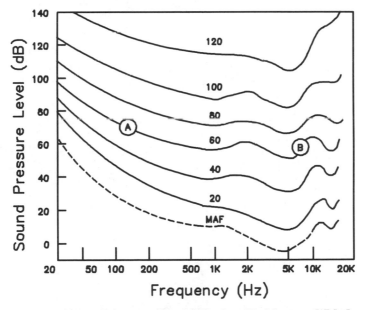

Figure 3.19. Equal-loudness contours from Fletcher H, Munson WN: Loudness, its definition, measurement, and calculation. *J Acoust Soc Am* 5:82–108, 1933. Each curve displays the combinations of frequency and intensity judged to be equal in loudness to a 1000-Hz tone having an SPL indicated above each contour. Point *A*, for example, indicates that a 125-Hz tone at 75 dB SPL is as loud as a 1000-Hz tone at 60 dB. (Note that frequency scale is logarithmic.) *MAF*, minimum audible field, or the threshold contour for free-field testing.

frequencies than at intermediate frequencies. It took only an 80-dB increase in sound level to go from a sound that was just audible (10 phons) to one that was uncomfortably loud (120 phons) at 100 Hz, whereas an increase of 110 dB was needed to cover this same range of loudness at 1000 Hz.

Another scale of loudness that has been developed, is the sone scale. The sone scale is derived by first defining the loudness of a 1000-Hz, 40-dB SPL pure tone as 1 sone. Next, the listener is asked to set the intensity of a second, comparison stimulus so that it produces a loudness sensation either one-half or twice that of the 1-sone standard stimulus. These intensities define the sound levels associated with ½ and 2 sones, respectively. This procedure is then repeated, with the sound having a loudness of either ½ or 2 sones serving as the new standard signal. Figure 3.20 illustrates the relationship between the increase of loudness in sones and the increase in sound intensity. Consistent with Stevens' law, described previously, we find that the loudness-growth function is a straight line, with the exception of intensities near threshold, when plotted on log-log coordinates. The slope of this line is 0.6, indicating that Stevens' law for loudness is: $L=kP^{0.6}$, where L is loudness, k is a constant, and P is sound pressure. Note that over the linear range of the function in Figure 3.20, a 10-dB increase in sound pressure level yields a doubling of loudness. That is, at 1000 Hz, an increase in sound pressure level from 40 to 50 dB SPL or from 80 to 90 dB SPL corresponds to a doubling of loudness.

The *dashed line* in Figure 3.20 illustrates a loudness-growth function obtained at 1000 Hz in the presence of a broad-band masking noise. The intersection of the x axis by the *dashed line* at 40 dB SPL indicates that the threshold has been elevated 40 dB (from 0 to 40 dB SPL) due to the masking noise. As intensity is increased slightly above threshold, comparison of the two functions indicates that the loudness of a 50-dB SPL tone is greater in the quiet condition (2 sones) than in the masked condition (0.2 sones). At higher intensities, however, the

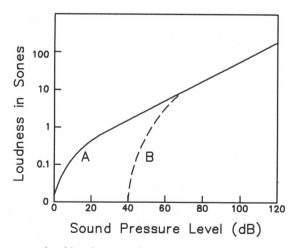

Figure 3.20. The growth of loudness with intensity in quiet (*A*) and in the presence of a background noise that produced 40 dB of masking (*B*). (Note that loudness scale is logarithmic.) Functions comparable to *B* are also obtained in hearing-impaired listeners having sensorineural hearing loss.

two functions merge, so that an 80-dB SPL tone has a loudness of 16 sones in both cases. Thus, in the masked condition, loudness grows very rapidly to "catch up" with the loudness perceived in the unmasked condition. This rapid growth of loudness is also a characteristic of ears that have a type of hearing loss known as sensorineural hearing loss, which affects the hair cells within the cochlea. The rapid growth of loudness in ears with sensorineural hearing loss is known as loudness recruitment. Its presence helps signify that the hearing loss is caused by pathology located within the cochlea. Unfortunately, loudness recruitment presents the audiologist with considerable difficulties in attempting to fit the patients who exhibit it with amplification devices, such as hearing aids. Low-level sounds must be amplified a specified amount to make them audible to the hearing-impaired listener. If high-level sounds are amplified by the same amount, however, they are uncomfortably loud, just as they would be in a normal ear.

Binaural Hearing

The final section of this chapter deals with the manner in which the information encoded by one ear interacts with that encoded by the other ear. The processing of sound by two ears is referred to as binaural hearing.

The localization of sound in space, for instance, is largely a binaural phenomenon. A sound originating on the right side of a listener, for example, will arrive first at the right ear because it is closer to the sound source. A short time later, the sound will reach the more distant left ear. This produces an interaural (between-ear) difference in the time of arrival of the sound at the two ears. The ear being stimulated first will signal the direction from which the sound arose. As might be expected, the magnitude of this interaural time difference will increase as the location of the sound source changes from straight ahead (called 0° azimuth) to straight out to the side (90° or 270° azimuth). As shown in Figure 3.21**A**, when the sound originates directly in front of the listener, the length of the path to both ears is the same, and there is no interaural difference in time of arrival of the sound. At the extreme right or left, however, the difference between the length of the path to the near ear and the length of the path to the far ear is greatest (and corresponds to the width of the head). This then will produce the maximum interaural time difference. Figure 3.21**B** illustrates the dependence of the interaural time difference on the azimuth of the sound source.

For frequencies below approximately 1500 Hz, the interaural time difference could also be encoded meaningfully into an interaural phase difference. From Figure 3.21**B**, for example, we see that at 60° azimuth an interaural time difference of approximately 0.5 ms results. This would occur for all frequencies. For a pure tone, however, one that completes 1 cycle in 1 ms (frequency=1000 Hz), this means that the signal to the far ear would be starting 0.5 cycle after the signal to the near ear. The two signals, therefore, would have a 180° phase difference between the two ears. A pure tone of 500 Hz having a 2-ms period and also originating from 60° azimuth, however, would only be delayed one-fourth of the period (0.5 ms/2.0 ms), corresponding to a 90° interaural phase difference. We see that, although interaural time differences are the same for all frequencies, the interaural phase differences resulting from these time differences vary with frequency.

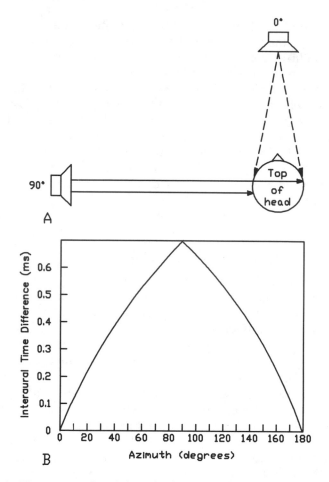

Figure 3.21. **A,** Illustration of path lengths from sound source to the left and right ears for 0° azimuth (*dashed lines*) and 90° azimuth (*solid lines*). **B,** Illustration of the interaural (between-ear) time differences as a function of azimuth for the spherical head assumed in **A.** At 0° and 180°, the sound arrives at the left and right ears simultaneously, resulting in no interaural time difference. The maximum interaural time difference occurs at 90°.

Interaural intensity differences are also produced when a sound originates from a location in space. These differences result from a sound shadow being cast by the head. Recall from Chapter 2 that, when the wavelength of the sound is small relative to the dimensions of the object, a sound shadow is produced. The magnitude of the sound shadow created by the head increases with frequency above 500 Hz. It produces interaural intensity differences of 20 dB at 6000 Hz for 90° or 270° azimuth. That is, the intensity of a 6000-Hz pure tone at the near ear is 20 dB greater than that measured at the far ear when the sound originates straight to the side of the listener (90° or 270° azimuth). At 500 Hz, the maximum interaural intensity difference is less than 4 dB. The interaural intensity difference decreases to 0 dB at all frequencies for 0° azimuth (straight ahead).

Thus, there are two primary acoustic cues for the localization of sound in space (specifically, the horizontal plane): interaural time differences and interaural intensity differences. The duplex theory of sound localization in the horizontal plane (left to right) maintains that both cues may be utilized over a wide range of frequencies by the listener in identifying the location of a sound source, but that interaural time differences predominate at low frequencies and interaural intensity differences at high frequencies. In contemporary theories of sound localization, several additional monaural and binaural cues are included, but interaural time and intensity differences are considered to be the strongest cues.

Masking is a topic that has also been explored in considerable detail in the binaural system. Experiments conducted in the late 1940s and the 1950s indicated that certain combinations of binaural signals and maskers could make the signal more detectable than others. Consider the following example. A noise masker and a pure-tone signal are presented equally and identically to both ears. The signal threshold is then determined. Then the pure-tone signal is removed from one ear, and the signal becomes easier to detect! This release from masking has been named the masking level difference (MLD) and corresponds to the change in threshold between two test conditions. The initial or reference threshold is usually determined for identical maskers and signals delivered to both ears. This is referred to as a diotic condition. Diotic stimulus presentations are those that deliver identical stimuli to both ears. Sometimes the reference threshold involves a masker and signal delivered to only one ear. This is called a monotic condition. After establishing the masked threshold in one of these reference conditions, the signal threshold is measured again under any one of several dichotic conditions. A dichotic test condition is one in which different stimuli are presented to the two ears. In the example described above, in which the signal was removed from one ear, the removal of the signal made that condition a dichotic one. That is, one ear received the masker and the pure-tone signal, while the other received only the masker. In general, a signal is more readily detected under dichotic masking conditions than under diotic or monotic masking conditions. For a given dichotic condition, the MLD is greatest at low frequencies (100–500 Hz), increases with the intensity of the masker, and is typically 12–15 dB under optimal stimulus conditions.

SUMMARY

In this chapter, we have reviewed the structure and function of the auditory system. The anatomy and physiology of the auditory system were discussed in the first portion. The amplification and impedance-matching functions of the outer and middle ear were reviewed. The importance of both a temporal or timing code and a place code (tonotopic organization) within the auditory system was emphasized. Perceptual phenomena, such as loudness and masking, were also reviewed, with an emphasis on those features of clinical relevance.

References and Suggested Readings

Durrant JD, Lovrinic JH: *Bases of Hearing Science*, ed 2. Baltimore, Williams & Wilkins, 1984.

Gelfand SA: *Hearing: An Introduction to Psychological and Physiological Acoustics.* New York, Marcel Dekker, 1981.

Humes LE: Psychoacoustic foundations of clinical audiology. In Katz J (ed): *Handbook of Clinical Audiology*, ed 3. Baltimore, Williams & Wilkins, 1985.

Møller AR: *Auditory Physiology.* New York, Academic Press, 1983.

Moore BCJ: *An Introduction to the Psychology of Hearing*, ed 2. London, Academic Press, 1982.

Pickles JO: *An Introduction to the Physiology of Hearing*, ed 2. London, Academic Press, 1988.
Shaw EAG: The external ear. In Keidel WD, Neff WD, (eds): *Handbook of Sensory Physiology*, vol V(1). New York, Springer Verlag, 1974, pp. 455–490.
von Bekesy G: *Experiments in Hearing*. New York, McGraw-Hill, 1960.
Wever EG, Lawrence M: *Physiological Acoustics*. Princeton, NJ, Princeton University Press, 1954.
Yost WA, Neilsen DW: *Fundamentals of Hearing: An Introduction*, ed 2. New York, Holt, Rinehart & Winston, 1985.
Zemlin WR: *Speech and Hearing Science: Anatomy and Physiology*, ed 2. Englewood Cliffs, NJ, Prentice-Hall, 1988.

PART TWO

ASSESSMENT OF AUDITORY FUNCTION

Chapter Four

Audiologic Measurement

The nature of auditory impairment is dependent on such factors as the severity of the hearing loss, the age at onset, the cause of the loss, and the location of the lesion within the auditory system. The hearing evaluation plays an important role in determining some of these factors. Audiometric measurement of auditory function can: (*a*) determine the degree of hearing loss; (*b*) estimate the location of the lesion within the auditory system that is producing the problem; (*c*) help establish the cause of the hearing problem; (*d*) estimate the extent of the handicap produced by the hearing loss; and (*e*) help to determine the client's habilitative or rehabilitative needs and the appropriate means of filling those needs. This chapter will focus on those tests used most commonly in the evaluation of auditory function. This battery of tests includes pure-tone audiometry, speech audiometry, and acoustic immittance measures.

OBJECTIVES

Following completion of this chapter, the reader should be able to:

- Understand the procedures for measuring pure-tone threshold by air conduction and by bone conduction.
- Understand the procedures for measuring hearing sensitivity for speech (speech-recognition threshold) and speech recognition.
- Identify situations requiring the use of contralateral masking and understand the concept of masking.
- Recognize the special modifications of these basic measurements needed for application to pediatric populations.
- Understand acoustic immittance measurements.
- Appreciate the way in which each test result represents just one aspect of the complete basic audiologic test battery.

CASE HISTORY

Before the audiologic evaluation begins, the audiologist obtains a history from the client. For adults, this history may be supplied by completing a printed form prior to the evaluation. The form contains pertinent identifying information for the client, such as home address, social security number, and referral source. Questions regarding the nature of past and present hearing problems, other medical problems, and prior use of amplification are also usually included. The written responses are then followed up during an interview between the audiologist and the client prior to any testing.

For children, the case history form is usually more comprehensive than the adult version. In addition to questions such as were mentioned for adults, detailed questions about the mother's pregnancy and the child's birth are included. The development of gross and fine motor skills and the development of speech and language are also probed. The medical history of the child is also reviewed in detail, with special emphasis on childhood diseases (measles, mumps, etc.) capable of producing a hearing loss. (See Chapter 5.)

PURE-TONE AUDIOMETRY

Pure-tone audiometry represents the basis of a hearing evaluation. With pure-tone audiometry, hearing thresholds are measured for pure tones at different test frequencies. Hearing threshold is typically defined as the lowest (softest) sound level needed for a person to detect the presence of a signal approximately 50% of the time. Threshold information at each frequency is then plotted on a graph known as an audiogram. Before examining the audiogram, however, we shall describe the equipment used to measure hearing.

The Audiometer

An audiometer is the primary instrument used by the audiologist to measure hearing threshold. Types of audiometers vary from the simple, inexpensive screening devices used in schools and public health programs to the more elaborate and expensive diagnostic audiometers found in hospitals and clinics. Certain basic components, however, are common to all audiometers. An example of one of these basic units is shown in Figure 4.1. A frequency selector dial provides for the selection of different pure-tone frequencies. Ordinarily these frequencies are available at octave intervals ranging from 125 to 8000 Hz. An interrupter switch or presentation button provides the capability of presenting the tone to the

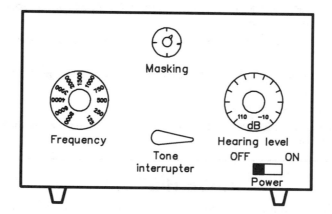

Figure 4.1.   Representation of the basic components seen on the control panel of a pure-tone audiometer.

listener. A hearing level dial controls the intensity of the signal. Most audiometers have the capacity to deliver signals spanning a 100-dB range in 5-dB steps. An output selector determines whether the pure tone will be presented to the earphones for air conduction testing (for either the right or left ear), or whether the tone is to be sent to a bone vibrator for bone conduction testing. Many audiometers also have a masking level dial, which controls the intensity of the masking noise presented to the nontest ear when masking is necessary. The more elaborate diagnostic audiometers not only can generate masking noise and pure-tone signals but also provide a means for measuring the understanding of speech signals.

The Audiogram

The audiogram is a chart used to record graphically the hearing thresholds and other test results. An example of an audiogram and the associated symbol system recommended by the American Speech-Language-Hearing Association is illustrated in Figure 4.2. The audiogram is shown in graphic form, with the signal frequencies (in Hertz) displayed on the *x* axis and hearing level (in decibels) represented on the *y* axis. The graph is designed in such a manner that 1 octave on the frequency scale is equal in size to 20 dB on the hearing level scale.

The horizontal line at 0 dB hearing level (HL) represents normal hearing

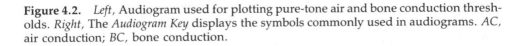

Figure 4.2. *Left,* Audiogram used for plotting pure-tone air and bone conduction thresholds. *Right,* The *Audiogram Key* displays the symbols commonly used in audiograms. *AC,* air conduction; *BC,* bone conduction.

sensitivity for the average young adult. However, as described in the previous chapter, the human ear does not perceive sound equally well at all frequencies. Recall that the ear is most sensitive to sound in the intermediate-frequency region from 1000 to 4000 Hz and is less sensitive at both the higher and lower frequencies. Greater sound pressure is needed to elicit a threshold response at 250 Hz than at 2000 Hz in normal ears. The audiometer is calibrated to correct for these differences in threshold sensitivity at various frequencies. Consequently, when the hearing level dial is set at zero for a given frequency, the signal is automatically presented at the normal threshold sound pressure level required for the average young adult to hear that particular frequency (Vignette 4.1).

Results plotted on the audiogram can be used to classify the extent of a hearing handicap. This information plays a valuable role in determining the habilitative or rehabilitative needs of a hearing-handicapped individual. Classification schemes using the pure-tone audiogram are based on the fact that there is a strong relationship between the threshold for those frequencies known to be important for hearing speech (500, 1000, and 2000 Hz) and the lowest level at which speech can be recognized accurately 50% of the time. The latter measure is generally referred to as the speech recognition threshold, or SRT. Given the pure-tone thresholds at 500, 1000, and 2000 Hz, the hearing loss for speech and the potential handicapping effects of the impairment can be estimated. This is done by simply calculating the average (mean) loss of hearing for these three frequencies. This average is referred to as the three-frequency pure-tone average. An example of a typical classification system based on the pure-tone average is shown in Figure 4.3. This scheme, adapted from several other systems, reflects the different classifications of hearing loss as well as the likely effects of the hearing loss on an individual's ability to hear speech. The hearing loss classes, ranging from mild to profound, are based on the pure-tone average at 500, 1000, and 2000 Hz. The classification of normal limits extends to 25 dB HL, and hearing levels within this range have typically been thought to produce essentially no problems with even faint speech. Some evidence indicates that losses from 15 to 25 dB HL, however, can have negative effects educationally on children.

Measurement of Hearing

In pure-tone audiometry, thresholds are obtained by both air conduction and bone conduction. In air conduction measurement, the different pure-tone stimuli are transmitted through earphones. The signal travels through the ear canal, across the middle ear cavity via the three ossicles to the cochlea, and on to the auditory central nervous system as reviewed in the previous chapter. Air conduction thresholds reflect the integrity of the total peripheral auditory mechanism. When a person exhibits a hearing loss by air conduction, it is not possible to determine where along the auditory pathway the pathology is located. The hearing loss could be the result of either: (*a*) a problem in the outer or middle ear; (*b*) a difficulty at the level of the cochlea; (*c*) damage along the neural pathways to the brain; or (*d*) some combination of (*a*), (*b*), or (*c*). When air conduction measurements are used in combination with bone conduction measurements, however, it is possible to differentiate between outer ear and middle ear problems (conductive hearing loss) and inner ear problems (sensorineural hearing loss).

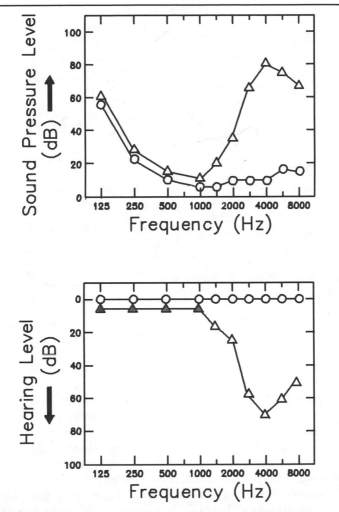

Vignette 4.1. Illustration of the Relationship between dB SPL and dB HL

The accompanying figure depicts the relationship between the dB HL scale and the dB SPL scale of sound intensity. The circles in the *upper panel* are the data for hearing thresholds of normal-hearing young adults. The triangles in the *upper panel* are hearing thresholds obtained from an individual with a high-frequency hearing loss. Note that increasing hearing loss is indicated by higher sound pressure levels at threshold. At 4000 Hz, for example, the average threshold for normal-hearing young adults is 10 dB SPL and the patient's threshold is 80 dB SPL, indicating a hearing loss of 70 dB. These same data have been replotted on the dB HL scale in the *lower panel*. Note now that the normal hearing threshold has been set to 0 dB HL on this scale at all frequencies. Increasing intensity is shown in a downward direction on the audiogram. Note also that the threshold for the hearing-impaired subject at 4000 Hz is 70 dB HL. This threshold value itself then directly indicates the magnitude of hearing loss relative to normal hearing. There is no need to subtract the normal-hearing threshold value from the value observed in the impaired ear, as was the case for the dB SPL scale.

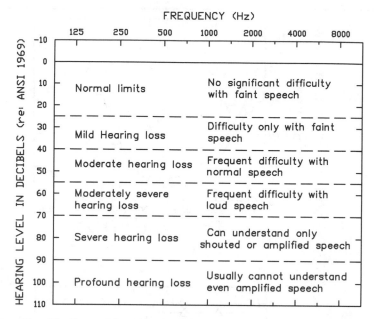

Figure 4.3.   Classification of hearing impairment in relation to handicap for speech recognition.

In bone conduction measurement, signals are transmitted by means of a bone vibrator that is usually placed on the mastoid prominence of the skull (a bony prominence located behind the pinna, slightly above the level of the concha). The forehead is another common position for placement of the bone vibrator. A signal transduced through the vibrator causes the skull to vibrate. The pure tone directly stimulates the cochlea, which is embedded in the skull, effectively bypassing the outer ear and middle ear systems. If an individual exhibits a reduction in hearing sensitivity when tested by air conduction yet shows normal sensitivity by bone conduction, the impairment is probably due to an obstruction or blockage of the outer or middle ear. This condition is referred to as a conductive hearing loss. An audiometric example of a young child with a conductive hearing loss due to middle ear disease is shown in Figure 4.4. The bone conduction thresholds (*[*, right-ear thresholds; *]*, left-ear thresholds) appear close to 0 dB HL for all test frequencies. Such a finding implies that the inner ear responds to sound at normal threshold levels. The air conduction thresholds (*0-0*, right ear; *X-X*, left ear), on the other hand, are much greater than 0 dB HL. Greater sound intensity is needed for this child to hear the air-conducted pure-tone signals than is required by the average normal hearer. Since the bone conduction thresholds suggest that the inner ear is normal, the loss displayed by air conduction must result from a conductive lesion affecting the outer or middle ear.

The difference between the air conduction threshold and the bone conduction threshold at a given frequency is generally referred to as the air-bone gap. In Figure 4.4, for example, at 250 Hz there is a 30-dB air-bone gap in the right ear and a 40-dB gap in the left ear. Conductive hearing loss is especially prevalent among preschool and young school-age children who experience repeated episodes of otitis media(middle ear infection). Other examples of pathologic condi-

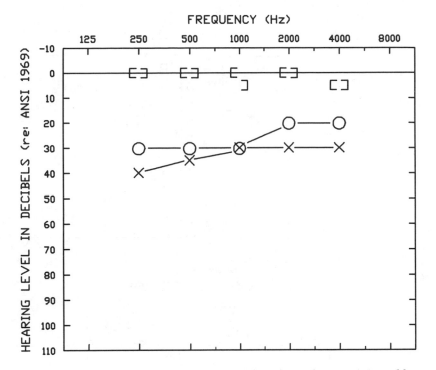

Figure 4.4. Pure-tone audiogram demonstrating the relation between air and bone conduction thresholds typifying mild conductive hearing impairment.

tions known to produce conductive hearing loss include congenital atresia (absence of ear canals), blockage or occlusion of the ear canal, perforation or scarring of the tympanic membrane, ossicular chain disruption, and otosclerosis. These pathologies are described in detail in Chapter 5.

As we noted, hearing thresholds better than a hearing level of 25 dB HL are considered normal. Air-bone gaps of 10 dB or more, however, represent a significant conductive hearing loss and may require medical referral, even if the air conduction thresholds are less than 25 dB at all frequencies.

A sensorineural hearing loss is suggested when the air conduction thresholds and bone conduction thresholds are approximately the same (± 5 dB) at all test frequencies. The cause of a sensorineural hearing impairment may be either congenital or acquired. Some of the congenital causes include heredity, complications of maternal viral and bacterial infections, and birth trauma. Factors producing acquired sensorineural hearing loss include noise, aging, inflammatory diseases (measles, mumps, etc.), and ototoxic drugs (e.g., aminoglycoside antibiotics). Many of these disorders are also described in Chapter 5. Three different examples of sensorineural hearing impairment are shown in Figure 4.5. Figure 4.5**A** represents the audiogram of an adult with a hearing loss resulting from the use of ototoxic antibiotics. This audiogram displays a moderate bilateral sensorineural impairment with a greater hearing loss in the high-frequency region. Figure 4.5**B** illustrates the audiogram of a child whose hearing impairment was the result of maternal rubella. It can be seen that the magnitude of this hearing loss falls in the profound category in the region of the most critical

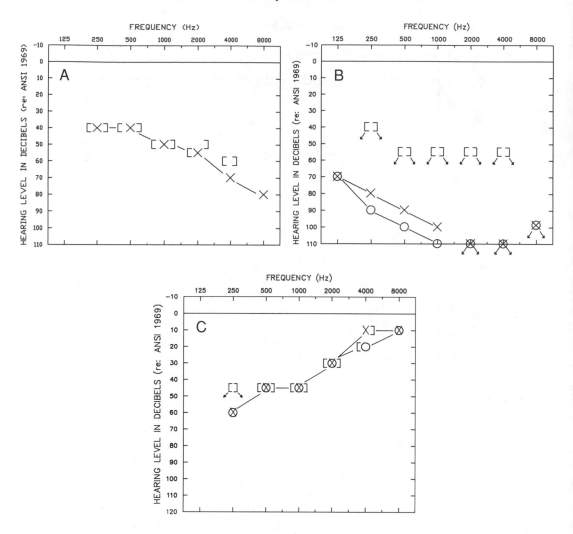

Figure 4.5. Three pure-tone air and bone conduction audiograms. **A,** Moderate bilateral sensorineural hearing loss. **B,** Profound bilateral sensorineural hearing loss. **C,** Low-frequency bilateral sensorineural hearing loss.

frequencies for hearing speech (500–2000 Hz). In fact, the loss is so severe that bone conduction responses could not be obtained at the maximum output of the audiometer at all test frequencies. This is indicated by the downward-pointing arrows attached to the audiometric symbols. Air conduction thresholds also could not be obtained at frequencies above 1000 Hz because the hearing loss was so great.

The majority of sensorineural hearing losses are characterized by audiometric configurations that are flat, trough shaped, or slightly to steeply sloping in the high frequencies. The latter is probably the most common configuration associated with acquired sensorineural hearing loss. Occasionally, however, patients display a sensorineural hearing loss in which the greatest hearing loss occurs at low and intermediate frequencies, with normal or near-normal hearing sensitivity at the high frequencies. An example of a typical low-frequency hearing loss is illustrated in Figure 4.5C. Low-tone hearing loss most commonly results from either some types of hereditary deafness or Ménière's disease. (See Chapter 5.) Young children whose audiograms display the low-frequency hearing impairment are difficult to identify and are sometimes the unfortunate victims of misdiagnosis. Because of their near-normal hearing sensitivity in the high frequencies, these children may respond to whispered speech and broad-band stimuli at low intensity levels. In addition, unlike children with a high-frequency hearing loss, their articulation of speech is usually good. These manifestations are not typical of sensorineural hearing loss in children, which makes them more prone to misdiagnosis.

When both air conduction thresholds and bone conduction thresholds are reduced in sensitivity, but bone conduction yields better results than air, the term mixed hearing loss is used. That is, the patient's hearing loss is partially conductive and partially sensorineural in nature. An example of mixed hearing loss is displayed in the audiogram shown in Figure 4.6. Even though hearing loss is evident for both bone and air conduction thresholds, bone conduction sensitivity is consistently better across all test frequencies. This suggests that there has been some damage to the hair cells or nerve endings in the inner ear, causing a reduction in bone conduction thresholds, which is added to the reduction in air conduction thresholds resulting from malfunction of the outer ear or middle ear.

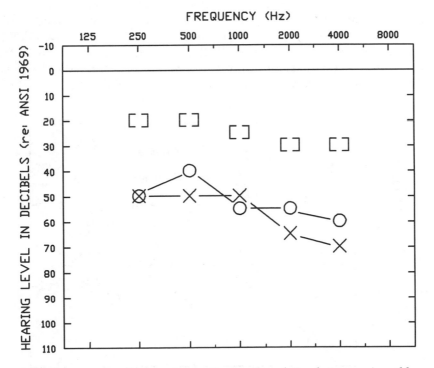

Figure 4.6. Pure-tone audiogram demonstrating the relation between air and bone conduction thresholds indicating a mixed (conductive and sensorineural) type of hearing loss.

Procedures for Obtaining Threshold

The hearing examination is generally conducted in a sound-treated room where noise levels are kept at a minimum and do not interfere with or influence the hearing test results. Pure-tone audiometry begins with air conduction measurements at octave intervals ranging from 125 or 250 Hz to 8000 Hz; these are followed by bone conduction measurements at octave intervals ranging from 250 to 4000 Hz. (Air conduction measurements at 125 Hz are optional. Some audiometers do not include this frequency.) The initial step in measuring threshold involves instructing the patient as to the listening and responding procedures. The listener is instructed to respond to the pure-tone signals no matter how soft they might be, to respond as soon as the tone is heard, and to stop responding when the sound becomes inaudible. The most common form of response is merely raising or lowering the forefinger. Earphones should be placed carefully and snugly on the patient's head so that the signal source is directed toward the opening of the ear canal.

Because 1000 Hz is considered to be the frequency most easily heard under headphones, and the threshold at this frequency is the most reliable, it is used as the initial test frequency and is administered first to the better ear. The right ear is tested first if the patient indicates that hearing sensitivity is the same in both ears. The most common procedure for establishing threshold is known as the ascending technique. An example of this pure-tone procedure is shown in Figure 4.7. An interrupted signal is presented at a hearing level of approximately 30 dB. If the listener is unable to perceive the tone at this level, the signal is then increased by 20 dB and presented again. This procedure is continued until the listener indicates that a signal has been perceived. For the case shown in Figure 4.7, the initial presentation level of 30 dB HL produced a response in the listener. After each positive response, the intensity dial setting is decreased in 10-dB steps until a hearing level is reached at which there is no response on the part of the

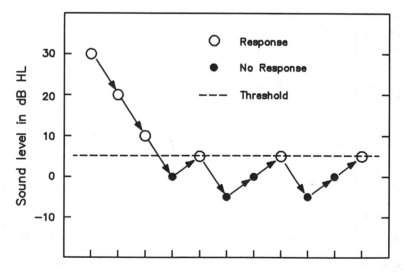

Figure 4.7. Alternating descending and ascending sound level presentations commonly used in obtaining pure-tone thresholds.

listener. Once the subject fails to respond to the signal, the actual ascending technique begins. Following a failure to obtain a response, the signal is increased in 5-dB increments until a response is obtained. Every time a positive response is obtained, the signal is decreased by 10 dB. As soon as the listener's response changes to no response, an ascending series of 5-dB steps is begun again. This process is continued until an intensity level used in an ascending series is found to which the listener responded positively at least 50% of the time. This level is then recorded as the threshold. In practice, if the listener responds at the same *ascending* level for two of two, two of three, two of four, or three of five presentations, this level is considered the threshold. Once this procedure has been completed at 1000 Hz, the examiner goes on to the higher test frequencies (2000, 4000, and 8000 Hz) and then returns to 1000 Hz for a reliability check. The lower frequencies, 500 and 250 Hz, are presented last. After testing all of the frequencies in one ear, the examiner then switches the signal to the opposite ear and repeats the procedures.

Essentially the same procedures are utilized for obtaining the bone conduction thresholds except that only frequencies from 250 through 4000 Hz are used. A bone vibrator is attached by a tension band to the mastoid prominence of the test ear or to the forehead so that the signal is transmitted via the bone pathways of the skull, bypassing the outer and middle ear. Once pure-tone thresholds have been completed using the same procedures as those described for air conduction, the bone vibrator, if placed on the mastoid prominence, is then removed and placed on the opposite mastoid prominence for completion of the bone conduction threshold measurements. If the bone vibrator is placed on the forehead, both inner ears can be evaluated from this location and there is no need to move the bone vibrator.

Factors That Can Influence Threshold

To ensure accurate threshold measurement, it is important to take every precaution to eliminate variables that can influence the threshold test. The following factors are known to be significant.

Proper Maintenance and Calibration of the Audiometer

Like all pieces of electronic equipment, the audiometer is subject to malfunction, especially with extensive usage. It is critical that the audiometer be handled carefully to ensure reliable results, and that it be checked electroacoustically and biologically (listening checks) on a periodic basis. Such services can usually be obtained at a university hearing clinic or at the manufacturer's distributorship.

Test Environment

Threshold measurement may also be affected if there are high ambient noise levels present at the time of the test. The evaluation should be conducted in a sound-treated environment designed specifically for hearing threshold measurement. If such facilities are not available, every precaution should be taken to perform the evaluation in the quietest room possible.

Earphone Placement

Inadequate positioning of the earphones can produce threshold errors as great as 10-15 dB. The audiologist should be sure that the tension band holding the earphones offers a snug yet comfortable fit and that the phones are placed carefully over the ear canal openings. The problems of earphone placement may be especially difficult with hyperactive children, very young children (under 2 years of age), or elderly adults. An alternative to conventional earphones is described in Vignette 4.2.

Placement of the Bone Vibrator

In testing for bone conduction, the vibrator is usually positioned on the prominence of the mastoid bone. Thresholds can vary, however, depending on the placement. To ensure the most accurate placement, it is advisable to introduce a comfortably loud pure tone at 1000 Hz and vary the position of the vibrator on the mastoid while asking the subject to report where the signal is loudest. With

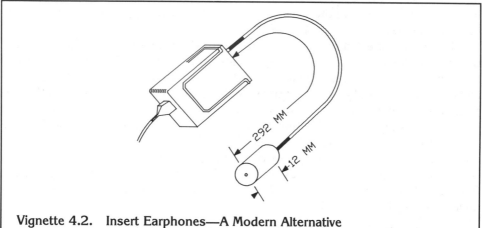

Vignette 4.2.   Insert Earphones—A Modern Alternative to Conventional Headphones

The drawing that accompanies this vignette illustrates a popular alternative to conventional headphones for testing hearing, known as *Tubephones*. As shown in the drawing, a long tube (292 mm in length) is used to conduct the sound from a pocket-sized electronic device to a soft cylindrical ear insert. The ear insert is a soft foam material that can be compressed temporarily by rolling it between the fingers. While it is compressed, it is inserted deeply into the ear canal and held in place for about 1 minute. This allows the foam material to expand and fit snugly in the ear canal. The pocket-sized electronic device is connected to the audiometer just like typical headphones. The *Tubephones* represent a special type of earphone known as insert earphones.

Insert earphones have become increasingly popular among audiologists for several reasons. When they are calibrated appropriately, the thresholds measured with them will be the same as those measured with conventional headphones. The insert phones also reduce the environmental noise levels more than conventional headphones. This enables them to be used in somewhat noisier test areas without the ambient noise affecting test results. The insert phones are also more comfortable to wear and fit children as well as they do adults. Finally, masking (discussed later in this chapter) is needed less frequently when testing by air conduction. At present, their primary disadvantage is cost, but this is likely to be less of a problem in the future.

younger children, such a practice may not be feasible, and special care must be taken to position the vibrator on a prominent portion of the mastoid bone.

The tension of the headband should also be checked on a periodic basis. After extensive use, the headbands for bone vibrators begin to lose tension and reduce the force that holds the vibrator against the mastoid process. Bone conduction thresholds are known to vary depending on the force applied to the vibrator. Again, because most tension bands were designed for adult-sized heads, special care must be taken when positioning the bone vibrator on the head of a child.

Procedures for Young Children

The procedures for pure-tone audiometry previously described represent those techniques recommended for older children and adults. Considerable modification of these techniques is required for testing the hearing of younger children. This section will focus on procedures used with infants and children between the ages of 2 months and 5 years.

Testing the Younger Infant, Aged 2 Months to 2 Years

A child between the ages of 2 months and 2 years is somewhat easier to evaluate than a newborn because the increased maturity results in more sophisticated and reliable responses. By approximately 3 months of age, attending responses are elicited easily and the infant is able to determine the location of the sound source in the horizontal plane. The audiologist's assessment of hearing in this age category is generally centered around behavioral observation conducted in a sound-field setting. An example of a typical test arrangement for sound-field audiometry is shown in Figure 4.8. The infant is placed in a high chair or on the mother's lap between two loudspeakers located at a 45° angle from both sides of the child. A controlled auditory signal is then presented at a level well above threshold (usually 50–85 dB HL), and behavioral responses are observed. The signal is decreased systematically in 10- to 20-dB steps for each positive response and increased 10 dB for each negative response. The nature of a positive response varies with the infant's age. Age-appropriate responses are discussed below. Threshold is usually defined as the lowest presentation level at which an infant responds 50% of the time. Some type of visual reinforcement is used to train the infant in the task and to reward the infant for responding appropriately.

The nature of the signal varies. Some clinicians favor the use of various noisemakers, such as a squeeze toy, bell, rattle, or spoon in a cup. While these signals are considered favorable in that they maintain a certain amount of interest on the part of the child and appear to be effective for eliciting arousal responses in young children or infants, they have inappropriate frequency characteristics. Most noisemakers contain energy at several frequencies. This makes it difficult to define the way in which the hearing loss varies with frequency and, in many cases, to determine if a hearing loss is present. If, for example, the infant has normal or near-normal hearing for low frequencies, the use of noisemakers that have energy at low and high frequencies will always produce a normal response in this infant even though a severe or profound high-frequency hearing loss might be present. If noisemakers are chosen as the test signal, the importance of

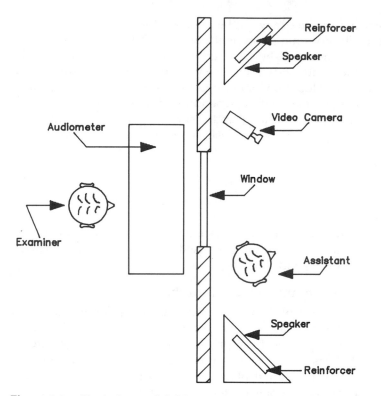

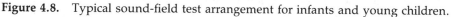

Figure 4.8. Typical sound-field test arrangement for infants and young children.

a careful acoustic analysis cannot be overemphasized. The clinician should be familiar with both the frequency and intensity characteristics of any noisemaker being used for hearing measurement. Most clinicians, however, favor the use of electronically generated signals such as narrow-band and complex noise, warble tones (tones that change slightly in frequency over time), and speech. With these types of test signals, the relevant stimulus parameters, such as intensity and frequency, can be carefully controlled and specified. Our clinical experience suggests that a combination of noisemakers, warble tones (frequency modulated) or noise, and filtered speech proves valuable in the hearing assessment of very young infants.

As mentioned, the kind of behavioral response produced by the young infant will vary depending on the child's age and the type of stimuli used. An index of the expected auditory response to various sounds for normal-hearing infants is shown in Table 4.1. The responses during the early months are typically arousal- or startle-oriented, whereas more sophisticated sound localization responses, such as head turns or eye movements in the direction of the loudspeaker producing the sound, occur with the older infants.

The use of a visual reinforcer in the measurement of hearing for very young infants is extremely important. Delivery of a visual stimulus following the appropriate sound-localization response serves to enhance the response behavior and leads to a more accurate threshold measurement. This technique is sometimes referred to as the conditioned orientation reflex (COR) or visual reinforcement

Table 4.1.
Index of Expected Auditory Responses to Various Sounds of Normal-Hearing Infants

Age	Stimulus			Expected Response
	Noisemakers (dB SPL)	Warbled Pure Tone[a,b] (dB HL)	Speech[a] (dB HL)	
Birth–6 weeks	50–70	78 (SD = 6)	40–60	Eye widening, eye blink, stirring or arousal from sleep, startle
6 weeks– 4 months	50–60	70 (SD = 10)	47 (SD = 2)	Eye widening, eye shift, eye blink, quieting; beginning rudimentary head turn by 4 months
4–7 months	40–50	51 (SD = 9)	21 (SD = 8)	Head turn on lateral plane toward sound; listening attitude
7–9 months	30–40	45 (SD = 15)	15 (SD = 7)	Direct localization of sounds to side, indirectly below ear level
9–13 months	25–35	38 (SD = 8)	8 (SD = 7)	Direct localization of sounds to side, directly below ear level, indirectly above ear level
13–16 months	25–30	32 (SD = 10)	5 (SD = 5)	Direct localization of sound on side, above, and below
16–21 months	25	25 (SD = 10)	5 (SD = 1)	Direct localization of sound on side, above, and below
21–24 months	25	26 (SD = 10)	3 (SD = 2)	Direct localization of sound on side, above, and below

[a]Adapted from Northern J, Downs M: *Hearing in Children*, ed. 3. Baltimore, Williams & Wilkins, 1984.
[b]SD, standard deviation.

audiometry (VRA). Visual reinforcers range from a simple blinking light to a more complex animated toy animal.

The scoring of a child's responses is also an important variable in the assessment of very young children. In order to assess sound localization behavior accurately, more than one person should observe the responses of the child. The clinician controlling the audiometer is very involved with the appropriate presentation of the auditory signals and can easily miss a behavioral response. It is desirable to have an assistant located in the examination room with the child to help in the scoring of responses.

There are limitations to sound-field audiometry performed with young infants. The most obvious limitations are: (*a*) the inability to obtain thresholds from each ear separately; (*b*) the inability to obtain bone conduction thresholds; and

(c) the failure to obtain responses from young children who have severe or profound hearing losses. The latter drawback results simply from the output limitations of typical audiometers when the sound is presented over loudspeakers. Sound-field testing has been considered the test of choice primarily because these children were considered too young to obtain valid earphone data.

Testing Children 2 to 5 Years Old

When the child reaches 2-5 years of age, he or she has matured sufficiently to permit more structured procedures to be used in the hearing evaluation. Those techniques used most frequently are conditioned play audiometry; tangible reinforcement operant conditioning audiometry (TROCA) or visual reinforcement operant conditioning audiometry (VROCA); and conventional (hand-raising) audiometry.

Conditioned play audiometry is the most well-accepted procedure for measuring the hearing thresholds of infants in this age group. The child participates in some form of play activity (e.g., placing a ring on a cone, putting blocks in a box, placing pegs in a hole) each time the signal is heard. The play activity serves as both the visible response for the clinician and the reinforcement for the child. Usually, social reinforcement also accompanies an appropriate response. The child is prevented from playing the game if an inappropriate response is made. The evaluation consists of a conditioning period in which the child is trained to perform the play activity in response to the delivery of a sound stimulus that is clearly audible. This is then followed by a threshold-seeking period. The technique may be employed in a sound-field condition or with earphone and bone conduction measurements. The application of play audiometry is limited to youngsters above the age of 2 years and those children who are not multiply handicapped.

Tangible reinforcement operant conditioning audiometry (TROCA) is a highly structured test procedure that was introduced originally as a means of assessing the hearing sensitivity of mentally retarded children. Although TROCA test procedures vary somewhat from clinic to clinic, the basic principle is that a tangible material, such as candy or trinkets (reinforcer), is automatically dispensed if the child depresses a button when a tone is perceived. If an inappropriate response is made, the child does not receive the reinforcement. TROCA incorporates specialized instrumentation that electromechanically controls the stimulus presentation, monitors the responses, and dispenses the tangible reinforcers. Like conditioned play audiometry, this technique may be employed either in a sound field or with earphone and bone conduction measurements. The use of TROCA has been extended from the mentally retarded population to young children, particularly those classified as difficult-to-test, such as distractible and hyperactive children. It is also considered useful when frequent retesting is required because reconditioning is seldom needed once the child is trained. The TROCA approach is not considered very successful with children below the age of 2½ years.

Visual reinforcement operant conditioning audiometry (VROCA) differs from TROCA only in that a visual reinforcement is used in place of a tangible reinforcer. Those who desire more detail on the audiometric procedures used with children should consult the appropriate suggested readings at the end of this chapter.

Masking

When hearing is assessed under earphones or with a bone vibrator, it is not always the case that the ear that the clinician desires to test is the one that is stimulated. Sometimes the other ear, referred to simply as the nontest ear, will be the ear stimulated by the sound. This situation results because the two ears are not completely isolated from one another. Air-conducted sound delivered to the test ear through conventional earphones mounted in typical ear cushions is decreased or attenuated approximately 40 dB before stimulating the other ear via skull vibration. The value of 40 dB for interaural ("between-ear") attenuation is actually a minimum value. The amount of interaural attenuation for air conduction varies with the frequency of the test signal but is always >40 dB. The minimum interaural attenuation value for bone conduction is 0 dB. Thus, the bone oscillator placed on the mastoid process behind the left ear vibrates the entire skull such that the effective stimulation of the right ear is essentially equivalent to that of the left ear. It is impossible, therefore, when testing by bone conduction, to discern whether the right ear or left ear is responding without some way of eliminating the participation of the nontest ear (Vignette 4.3).

Masking enables the clinician to eliminate the nontest ear from participation in the measurement of hearing thresholds for the test ear. Essentially, the audiologist introduces a sufficient amount of masking noise into the nontest ear so as to make any sound crossing the skull from the test ear inaudible.

There are two simple rules the audiologist follows in deciding whether to mask the nontest ear; one applies to air conduction testing and the other to bone conduction measurements. Regarding air conduction thresholds, masking is required at a given frequency if the air conduction threshold of the test ear exceeds the bone conduction threshold of the nontest ear by more than 35 dB. Recall that the bone conduction threshold may be equivalent to or better than the air conduction threshold but never poorer. Thus, if one observes a 50-dB difference between the air conduction thresholds of the two ears at a particular frequency, the difference will be *at least* that great when the comparison is made between the air conduction threshold of the test ear and the bone conduction threshold of the nontest ear. Consequently, one need not always determine the bone conduction threshold of the nontest ear prior to reaching a decision regarding masking for air conduction. This is made more clear with the following example. The patient indicates that hearing is better in the right ear, and air conduction testing is initiated with that ear. A threshold of 10 dB HL is observed at 1000 Hz. Following completion of testing at other frequencies in the right ear, the left ear is tested. An air conduction threshold of 50 dB HL is observed at 1000 Hz. Is this an accurate indication of the hearing loss at 1000 Hz in the left ear? The audiologist can't be sure. The air conduction threshold for the right ear is 10 dB HL and indicates that the bone conduction threshold for that ear at 1000 Hz is not greater than this value. Thus, there is *at least* a 40-dB difference between the air conduction threshold of the test ear at 1000 Hz (50 dB HL) and the bone conduction threshold of the nontest ear (≤ 10 dB HL). If the skull only attenuates

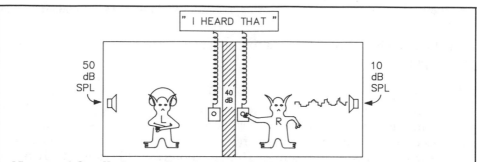

Vignette 4.3. Understanding the Need for Masking

In the drawing that accompanies this vignette, two gremlins named "Lefty" and "Righty" are shown, one in each of the two adjacent rooms. The two rooms are separated by a wall that decreases sound intensity by 40 dB. The gremlins' job is to listen for pure tones in their rooms. When they hear a sound, they are to signal by pushing a button to light a neon sign containing the words "I heard that!" In the illustration above, Righty hears a 10-dB SPL sound coming from the loudspeaker in his room and presses the button. By using softer and louder intensities, we determine the sound intensity that Righty responds to 50% of the time and call this his threshold. Righty has a threshold of 10 dB SPL. This is the typical or normal threshold for most gremlins.

Next, we proceed to measure the hearing threshold of Lefty. Unbeknownst to us, Lefty has decided to cover his ears with earmuffs! (You have to be careful with gremlins!) The earmuffs reduce the sound reaching his ears by 60 dB! As we try to measure Lefty's threshold, we gradually increase the intensity of the sound coming from the loudspeaker in the left room. Finally, we get a response. About 50% of the time, we see the neon light flash above the rooms when the presentation level of the sound is 50 dB SPL. We conclude the Lefty's threshold is 50 dB SPL.

Is our conclusion correct? Probably not. We said that the earmuffs decrease the sound reaching Lefty's ears by 60 dB and that the typical threshold for gremlins is 10 dB SPL. If the sound level from the speaker in the left room is 50 dB SPL and the earmuffs decrease it by 60 dB, then the sound level reaching Lefty's ears is −10 dB SPL. This is well below threshold for gremlins! Yet, we clearly saw the neon light flash 50% of the time when the left speaker presented a sound level of 50 dB SPL. By now you have probably discovered that it was Righty responding to the sound from the left speaker, not Lefty. The wall decreases sound by 40 dB. A 50-dB SPL sound from the left speaker will be 10 dB SPL, in the right room. Righty's threshold is 10 dB SPL, and he responds accordingly by pushing the button and lighting the neon sign. Whenever the sound level presented to one room is 40 dB or more above the threshold of the gremlin in the other room, we can't be sure which gremlin is turning on the neon light.

If we used the loudspeaker in Righty's room to present a noise loud enough to make Righty's threshold higher than 10 dB SPL, we could then proceed to increase the sound from the left speaker above levels of 50 dB SPL. By introducing enough masking noise into Righty's room, we could eventually measure Lefty's real threshold of 70 dB SPL (10 dB SPL normal threshold plus 60 dB from earmuffs).

The gremlins in the drawing are like our inner ears and the loudspeaker like the headphones. The wall of 40 dB is the separation between the ears provided by the skull, known as the interaural (between-ear) attenuation. Masking noise is needed to determine which ear is really responding to sound.

the air-conducted sound delivered to the test ear by 40 dB, then a signal level of approximately 10 dB HL reaches the nontest ear. The level of the crossed-over signal approximates the bone conduction threshold of the nontest ear and may, therefore, be detected by that ear. Now assume that a masking noise is introduced into the nontest ear to raise that ear's threshold to 30 dB HL. If the air-conduction threshold of the test ear remains at 50–55 dB HL, we may safely conclude that the observed threshold provides an accurate indication of the hearing loss in that ear.

When testing hearing by bone conduction, masking is needed whenever the difference between the air conduction threshold of the test ear and the bone conduction threshold of the test ear at the same frequency (the air-bone gap) is $\geq$ 10 dB. Because the interaural attenuation for bone conduction testing is 0 dB, the bone conduction threshold is always determined by the ear having the better bone conduction hearing. Consider the following example. Air conduction thresholds obtained from both ears reveal a hearing loss of 30 dB across all frequencies in the left ear, while thresholds of 0 dB HL are obtained at all frequencies in the right ear. Bone conduction testing of each ear indicates thresholds of 0 dB HL at all frequencies. Is the 30-dB air-bone gap observed in the left ear a real indication of a conductive hearing loss in that ear? Without the use of masking in the measurement of the bone conduction thresholds of the left ear, the clinician can't answer that question confidently. We know that the bone conduction thresholds of the nontest ear (right) will be less than or equal to the air conduction threshold of that ear (0 dB HL). Thus, when we observe this same bone conduction threshold when testing the test ear (left), either of two explanations is possible. First, the bone conduction threshold could be providing a valid indication of the bone conduction hearing in that ear. This means that a conductive hearing loss is present in that ear. Second, the bone conduction threshold of the test ear could actually be poorer than 0 dB HL, but it could simply be reflecting the response of the better ear (the nontest ear with a threshold of 0 dB HL). By masking the nontest ear, we can decide between these two explanations for the observed bone conduction threshold of the test ear. If the bone conduction threshold of the test ear remains unchanged when sufficient masking noise is introduced into the nontest ear, we may safely conclude that it provides an accurate indication of bone conduction hearing in that ear.

As we have seen, the need to mask the nontest ear and the rules for when to mask are relatively straightforward. There are a variety of masking procedures that have been developed to determine how much masking is sufficient. A detailed description of these procedures is beyond the scope of this introductory text. A brief description of one particular approach, the plateau method, has been provided in the supplement at the end of this chapter. Additional references on masking can be found at the end of this chapter.

SPEECH AUDIOMETRY

Although pure-tone thresholds tell us much about the function of the auditory system, they do not provide the audiologist with a precise measure of a person's ability to understand speech. Speech audiometry, a technique designed to assess a person's ability to hear and understand speech, has become a basic tool in the overall assessment of hearing handicap. In this section, some of the applications of speech audiometry in the basic hearing evaluation will be reviewed.

The Speech Audiometer

Speech audiometry generally requires a two-room testing suite—a control room, which contains the audiometric equipment as well as the audiologist, and an evaluation room where the patient is located (Fig. 4.9). Most diagnostic audiometers include the appropriate circuitry for both pure-tone measurement and speech audiometric evaluation. The speech circuitry portion of a diagnostic audiometer consists of a calibrated amplifying system having a variety of options for input and output of speech signals. Most commonly, the speech audiometer accommodates inputs for a microphone, tape recorder, and phonograph. It is possible to conduct speech testing using "live" speech (microphone) or prerecorded materials. The output of the speech signal may be directed to earphones, a bone vibrator, or a loudspeaker situated in the test room. Speech-audiometric testing via air conduction can be conducted in one ear (monaurally), in both ears (binaurally), or in a sound-field environment. Bone conduction testing is also possible. Many diagnostic audiometers employ a dual-channel system that enables the examiner to incorporate two inputs at the same time and to direct these signals to any of the available outputs.

To ensure valid and reliable measurements, just as with pure-tone audiometry, the circuitry of the speech audiometer must be calibrated on a regular basis. The acoustic output of the speech audiometer is calibrated in dB relative to normal hearing threshold (dB HL). According to our most recent standards for speech audiometers, 0 dB HL is equivalent to 20 dB SPL when measured through earphones. There is a difference of approximately 7.5 dB between earphone and sound-field threshold measurements for speech signals. Consequently, 0 dB HL in the sound field corresponds to an output from a loudspeaker of approximately 12 dB SPL. This calculated difference in audiometric zero for earphones and

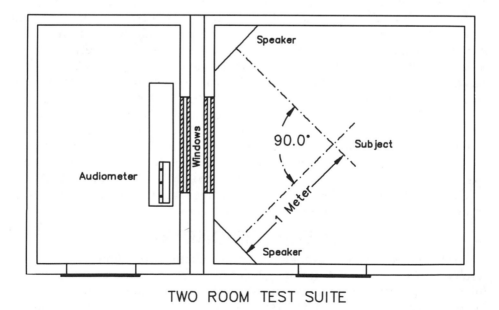

TWO ROOM TEST SUITE

Figure 4.9. Typical two-room test setup for speech audiometry.

loudspeakers makes it possible for us to obtain equivalent speech thresholds in dB HL under these two listening conditions.

Assessment of Speech-Recognition Threshold

Speech-recognition threshold (SRT) is the intensity at which an individual is able to identify simple speech materials approximately 50% of the time. It is included in the basic hearing evaluation for two specific reasons. First, it serves as an excellent check on the validity of pure-tone thresholds. There is a strong correlation between the average of the pure-tone thresholds obtained at the frequencies known to be important for speech (i.e., 500, 1000, and 2000 Hz) and the SRT. Large discrepancies between the SRT and this pure-tone average (PTA) may be suggestive of functional, or nonorganic, hearing loss. A second important reason for including the SRT in the hearing evaluation is that it provides a basis for selecting the sound level at which a patient's speech-recognition abilities should be tested. Finally, an important application of the SRT, beyond that of the basic hearing evaluation, is the determination of functional gain in the hearing aid evaluation process. (See Chapter 7.)

Speech-Threshold Materials

The most popular test materials used by audiologists to measure SRT are spondaic words. Spondaic words are two-syllable words spoken with equal stress on each syllable (e.g., baseball, hotdog, cowboy). A carrier phrase, such as "say the word," may precede each stimulus item. The spondaic words used most widely by audiologists are taken from the Central Institute for the Deaf (CID) Auditory Test W-1.

Speech-Threshold Procedures

Several different procedures have been advocated for determining the speech-recognition threshold utilizing spondaic words. The Committee on Audiometric Guidelines of the American Speech-Language-Hearing Association has recently revised its recommended test protocol. The recommended procedure uses most of the 36 spondaic words from the CID W-1 word list. The testing begins by first presenting all of the spondaic words to the client at a comfortable level. This familiarizes the patient with the words to be used in the measurement of threshold.

The actual test procedure is a descending threshold technique that consists of two phases: a preliminary phase and a test phase. In the preliminary phase, the first spondaic word is presented at 30–40 dB above the estimated threshold (pure-tone average) or at 50 dB HL, if an estimate can not be obtained. If the client fails to respond at this level or responds incorrectly, the starting level is increased 20 dB. This is continued until a correct response is obtained. A correct response is then followed by a 10-dB decrease in level until the response changes to an incorrect one. At this level, a second spondee is then presented. The level is decreased in 10-dB steps until two consecutive words have been missed at the same level. The level is then increased 10 dB above the level at which two consecutive spondees were missed. This represents the starting level for the next phase, the test phase.

During the test phase, two spondaic words are presented at the starting level and at each successive 2-dB decrement in level. If five of the first six spondees are repeated correctly, this process continues until five of the last six spondees are responded to incorrectly. If five of the first six stimuli were not repeated correctly, then the starting level is increased 4–10 dB and the descending series of stimulus presentations is initiated.

The descending procedure recommended by ASHA begins with speech levels above threshold and "descends" toward threshold. At the first few presentation levels, about 80% (5 of 6) of the items are correct. At the ending level, about 20% (1 of 6) spondees are repeated correctly. A formula is used to then calculate the SRT. The SRT represents the lowest hearing level at which an individual can recognize 50% of the speech material.

Assessment of Suprathreshold Speech Recognition

While the speech threshold provides the clinician with the index of the degree of hearing loss for speech, it does not offer any information regarding a person's ability to make distinctions among the various acoustic cues in our spoken language at conversational intensity levels. Unlike the situation with the SRT, attempts to calculate a person's ability to understand speech presented at comfortably loud levels based on data from the pure-tone audiogram have not been successful. Consequently, various suprathreshold speech-recognition tests have been developed for the purpose of estimating a person's ability to understand conversational speech. Three of the more common forms of speech-recognition testing include phonetically balanced word lists, multiple-choice tests, and sentence tests.

Phonetically Balanced Word Lists

The most popular phonetically balanced (PB) word lists are summarized in the top portion of Table 4.2. These word lists are referred to as "phonetically balanced" in that the phonetic composition of all lists are equivalent and representative of everyday English speech. All of the phonetically balanced word lists utilize an open-set response format. The listener is not presented with a closed set of several alternatives for each test item, one of which is the monosyllabic

Table 4.2.
A Summary of the Features of Several Common Speech-Recognition Tests

Response Format	Test	No. of Items (Alt.)[a]	No. of Lists[b]	Reference
Open	PAL PB-50	50	20	Egan (1)
	CID W-22	50	4	Hirsh et al. (2)
	NU #6	50	4	Tillman and Carhart (3)
Closed	MRHT	50 (6)	6	House et al. (4)
	CCT	100 (4)	2	Owens and Schubert (5)
	CUNY NST	67–102 (7–9)	1[c]	Levitt and Resnick (6)

[a]Alt., number of alternatives in the multiple-choice, closed response-set tests.
[b]Lists refer to sets of unique words.
[c]Although the same nonsense syllables are used, there are 14 randomizations of these materials available, seven with a female talker and seven with a male talker.

word spoken by the examiner. Rather, the set of possible responses to a test item is open and is limited only by the listener's vocabulary.

For comparison purposes, representative performance-intensity functions for many of these lists appear in Figure 4.10. As evidenced by Figure 4.10, a performance-intensity function describes performance (for either a group or an individual) in percent-correct recognition of the test items as a function of the intensity of the speech signal. The intensity of the speech signal is usually specified in dB above SRT (i.e., dB sensation level re: SRT, abbreviated dB SL). Because of their widespread use, performance on two different recordings of one set of items, the *CID W-22* lists, is illustrated in Figure 4.10. This figure readily demonstrates that differences do exist among the tests. The most difficult test among these monosyllabic materials is the PAL PB-50s. On the most linear portion of the curve (from 20 to 80% correct), identification performance for this test increases at a rate of 3.8%/dB. It is of interest to note the differences observed between the functions of the two recorded versions of the CID W-22s (labeled 3 and 5 in Fig. 4.10). Results for the most recent recording (5) are displaced to higher sensation levels than results for the original version (3). Such differences illustrate clearly that two different recordings of the same material can yield significantly different performance functions. It is the recorded words that comprise the test and not simply the printed list of words.

Multiple-Choice Tests

Some clinicians, unsatisfied with the conventional open-set PB words, directed their attention to alternative test formats for word-recognition testing. The

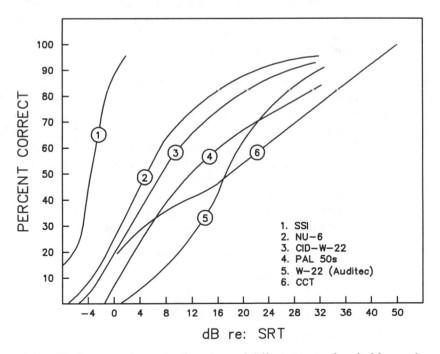

Figure 4.10. Performance-intensity functions of different suprathreshold speech-recognition tests. Functions 3 and 5 represent two different recordings of the W-22 material.

closed-set format inherent with multiple-choice tests was one of the most popular alternatives developed. The closed-set tests provide several advantages over open-set word-recognition tests. The closed-set format eliminates the need to familiarize a subject with the test vocabulary and reduces the potential for a practice effect. Other advantages of the closed-set format include elimination of examiner bias, ease of administration, and simplified scoring techniques.

The features of several popular multiple-choice tests are summarized in Table 4.2. The most widely recognized multiple-choice test, the Modified Rhyme Hearing Test (MRHT), was introduced in 1968 as a recorded clinical test of speech recognition by a group from the Stanford Research Institute. A sample test ensemble is shown in Figure 4.11. In this and other multiple-choice tests, the choices available to the listener usually differ from one another by only one speech sound.

A more recent development in multiple-choice tests has been the introduction of the California Consonant Test (CCT), a consonant-identification test developed for and standardized on a hearing-impaired population. The CCT is composed of two different scramblings of 100 test items, each of which is arranged within an ensemble of four consonant-vowel-consonant (CVC)monosyllabic words. For each item, the words are assembled so that either the initial two phonemes are the same, with the final varying, or, conversely, the final two phonemes are the same, with the initial phoneme varying. Of the 100 test items, 36 consonants are located in the initial position, whereas 64 consonants are found in the final position. An example consisting of four different test ensembles is shown in Figure 4.12.

The performance-intensity function for the CCT (labeled 6) is displayed in Figure 4.10. It is seen that the function for the CCT is distinctively different from the functions for the other test materials. The slope of the function is only 1.6%/dB. In addition, notice that maximum intelligibility is not reached until signal intensity reaches 50 dB SL (re: SRT).

Another recent development in speech audiometry is the emergence of closed-set nonsense syllable tests. One such test, the City University of New York (CUNY) Nonsense Syllable Test (NST), is composed of consonant-vowel and vowel-consonant syllables categorized into 11 subtests of seven to nine syllables each. The syllables in these subtests differ in: (*a*) consonant voicing (voiced or voiceless); (*b*) syllable position of the consonant (initial or final position); and (*c*) vowel context (/a, u, i/). An advantage of this test is that it is possible to analyze errors with respect to place and/or manner of articulation. With this test, it is possible to obtain a somewhat detailed picture of the *type* of errors made by the listener and not just an indication of the total number of errors made.

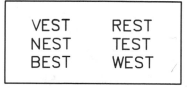

Figure 4.11.   Examples of a test ensemble used in the Modified Rhyme Hearing Test (MRHT).

```
BACK      _____    GAVE      _____
BAT       _____    GAME      _____
BATCH     _____    GAZE      _____
BATH      _____    GAGE      _____


THIN      _____    LEASE     _____
TIN       _____    LEASH     _____
SIN       _____    LEAF      _____
SHIN      _____    LEAP      _____
```

Figure 4.12.   Examples of four different test ensembles used in the California Consonant Test (CCT).

Sentence Tests

In an attempt to approximate everyday speech more closely, several speech identification tests have been developed using sentences as the basic test item. An advantage of speech tests using sentence materials over other types of speech tests is that sentences approximate the spectral and contextual characteristics of connected discourse while controlling for sentence length and semantic content. This increases the test's face validity.

The first sentence test designed for the clinical purpose of assessing speech recognition ability was developed and recorded at the Central Institute for the Deaf (CID). At present, however, there are no commercial recordings of these materials. Consequently, the clinical application of the CID sentences is somewhat limited.

One popular sentence test is the Synthetic Sentence Identification (SSI) test. The sentences used in this test were constructed such that each successive group of three words in the sentence was itself meaningful but the entire sentence was not. The following is an example of a test item from the SSI: "Forward march said the boy had a."

A sample performance-intensity function for the SSI is displayed in Figure 4.10. It is readily seen that this test is much easier than other materials shown in this figure. In an effort to increase the difficulty of this test, a competing speech message was mixed with the sentences. For clinical evaluation purposes, it was recommended that the SSI be administered at a message-to-competition ratio (MCR) of 0 dB; that is, both the speech and the competition are delivered at the same intensity level. This amount of competition provided performance scores in normal listeners which were comparable to scores obtained with phonetically balanced materials in a quiet environment.

Another sentence identification test, referred to as the SPIN (Speech Perception in Noise) test, has been developed recently. The eight available lists of the revised SPIN test are each composed of 50 sentences, each being five to eight words in length. The last word of each sentence is the test item. Twenty-five of the sentences contain test items that are classified as having "high predictability," which means that the word is readily predictable given the context of the sentence. Conversely, 25 sentences have test items with "low predictability." An example of a sentence containing a "high predictability" test item is:"The boat sailed across the *bay*," whereas an example of a sentence with "low predictability" using the same test word is: "John was talking about the *bay*." A recording of a background of babble-type competition composed of 12 voices reading simultaneously is also provided separately by the test's developers.

Speech Materials for the Pediatric Population

In this section, some speech materials commonly used to assess the word-recognition skills of children are reviewed. The major modification required in the evaluation of children is to ensure that the speech material is within the receptive vocabulary of the child under test. The required response, moreover, must be appropriate for the age tested. It would not be appropriate, for example, to ask for written responses from a 4-year-old on a word-recognition task!

The three most popular tests for use with the pediatric population are: (*a*) the Phonetically Balanced Kindergarten test (PBK-50s); (*b*) the Word Intelligibility by Picture Identification (WIPI) test; and (*c*) the Northwestern University Auditory Test No. 6 (NU-6). The performance-intensity function for the latter test was described previously in this chapter. The NU-6 materials are appropriate for use with adults and children 8 years of age and older. The PBK-50s, an open-response test, appears to be most suitable for children between the ages of 5 and 7 years.

For many younger children, the open-response design of the PBK-50s and NU-6s provides a complicated task, which causes difficulty in the administration and scoring of the test. For example, a child with a speech problem is difficult to evaluate because oral responses may not represent what the child actually perceived. In addition, children sometimes lose interest in the task because of the tedium associated with this type of format. Many children's lists have incorporated a closed-set response format as a means of minimizing some of the above problems.

Probably the most popular multiple-choice test for use with hearing-impaired children is the WIPI test. This test consists of four 25-word lists of monosyllabic words within the vocabulary of preschool-age children. For a given test item, the child is presented with a page containing six pictures, one of which is a pictorialization of the test item. The appropriate response of the child is to point to or touch the picture corresponding to the word perceived. The WIPI test is most appropriate for children between the ages of 2½ and 6 years.

Clinical Decisions in the Assessment of Speech Recognition

The speech recognition score can be influenced (sometimes to a large extent) by several variables, most of which are related to the procedures used in test administration. Because of their important implications for the audiologist, several of these variables are considered below.

Mode of Test Presentation

The audiologist needs to give thought to the details of test presentation. Speech-recognition scores can be affected dramatically by speaker differences, methods used in recording the test materials, and characteristics of the test equipment. When considering the protocol for presenting the test materials, there seem to be three issues that are of special concern to the clinician: (*a*) whether to use recorded materials or to employ a monitored live-voice presentation; (*b*) whether to utilize a carrier phrase; and (*c*) how to determine the appropriate intensity level at which to administer the test materials.

Generally, recorded materials offer greater test reliability than monitored live-voice presentations. The score on retest is more similar to previous results obtained just prior to retest when recorded materials are used. With many clinical populations, however, greater flexibility is needed than is offered by a tape-recorded test. This is frequently the case, for example, when testing young children. Under these circumstances, monitored live-voice presentation is preferred.

A common practice in the assessment of speech recognition is to preface each test item with a carrier phrase such as "Say the word _____," "You will say _____," or "Write the word _____." Carrier phrases are used for two basic purposes. First, they prepare the listener for the upcoming stimulus item, and second, they help the clinician monitor the intensity of the speech signal during monitored live-voice presentation.

Another important consideration for the audiologist is determining the intensity level that is most appropriate for administering a speech-recognition test. The objective is usually to estimate the listener's maximum ability to understand speech, often referred to as the "PB-max" when phonetically balanced monosyllabic materials are used. The only true means of obtaining the best speech-recognition score is to obtain a complete performance-intensity function. That is, several lists should be presented at successively higher intensity levels. Such a procedure, however, is clinically impractical because of the time required. Instead, clinicians attempt to estimate maximum speech-recognition ability from just one intensity level, usually 40 dB above the speech-recognition threshold. The intensity needed to yield a maximum recognition score will vary depending on the test material to be used. The variation in scores which may occur as a function of material was illustrated previously in Figure 4.10. It is noted, for example, that when using the CCT an intensity of 50 dB SL is required to achieve a maximum score, whereas with the original recordings of the W-22 materials, only 25 dB SL is needed to reach a best score.

Ideally, it is recommended that the clinician administer the speech-recognition test at two or three successively higher intensity levels, if time permits. Understandably, however, such a practice is simply not always practical in the clinical milieu. Sometimes the clinician will have to select one intensity level for estimating the PB-max.

Mode of Response

In scoring the responses to a speech-recognition test, the most common practice is for the clinician to judge whether the listener's oral response was correct or in error. However, if the patient is able, and if time permits, a written response should be employed in an effort to minimize any biases of the clinician. The patient's written responses are much easier to implement for multiple-choice tests.

Listening Conditions

There are limitations associated with the assessment of speech-recognition ability in a quiet environment. First, it is known that many of the available speech-recognition tests fail to differentiate among hearing-impaired listeners when administered in a quiet test condition. That is, the tests simply do not appear difficult enough to identify the problems experienced by many listeners with hearing loss. A second disadvantage with performing speech audiometry in quiet is that such a testing condition does not reflect the typical environment encountered in everyday listening situations.

In an attempt to increase the difficulty of the identification task and simulate a more realistic listening environment, audiologists have turned to the use of various types of background noises and competing messages in the assessment of speech recognition. In 1968, Carhart emphasized the need for clinicians to assess speech-recognition ability under conditions that more closely approximated typical listening situations. Carhart's impressions on this subject can best be summarized by his statement, ". . . once we have developed good methods for measuring a patient's capacity to understand speech under adverse listening conditions we will possess the audiological tools for dealing much more insightfully with his everyday listening problems" (7). Unfortunately, there are no standardized procedures, to date, for assessing recognition under adverse listening conditions, even though there is an abundance of literature in this area.

Several types of background noises or competition have been used in speech-recognition tests, including white noise, filtered and shaped noise, modulated white noise, cafeteria noise, and spoken messages (from one to several talkers). All such background signals are known to degrade the perception of the speech signal to various degrees. Unfortunately, the addition of background noise also increases the variability of test results and reduces the reliability of the data. Nonetheless, by measuring recognition under adverse listening conditions the clinician is able to assess more adequately the communicative handicap imposed by the patient's hearing impairment.

Masking

In speech audiometry, just as in pure-tone measurements, there exists the possibility of crossover from the test ear to the nontest ear. Consequently, when the level of the speech signal presented to the test ear exceeds the bone conduction threshold of the nontest ear, masking is necessary.

ACOUSTIC IMMITTANCE MEASUREMENT

Impedance, as mentioned in Chapter 2, is defined as the opposition to the flow of energy through a system. When an acoustic wave strikes the eardrum of the normal ear, a portion of the signal is transmitted through the middle ear to the cochlea, while the remaining part of the wave is reflected back out the external canal. The reflected energy forms a sound wave traveling in an outward direction with an amplitude and phase that is dependent upon the opposition encountered at the tympanic membrane. The energy of the reflected wave is greatest when the middle ear system is stiff or immobile, as in such pathologic conditions as otitis media with effusion, or otosclerosis. On the other hand, an ear with ossicular-chain interruption will reflect considerably less sound back into the canal because of the reduced stiffness. A greater portion of the acoustic wave will be transmitted to the middle ear under these circumstances. The reflected sound wave, therefore, carries information about the status of the middle ear system.

The reciprocal of impedance is admittance. An ear having a high impedance has a low admittance, and vice versa. Admittance describes the relative ease with which energy flows through a system. Some commercially available devices used by the clinician measure quantities related to acoustic impedance of the middle ear, while others measure quantities related to acoustic admittance. In an effort to provide a common vocabulary for results obtained with either device, professionals have decided to use the term immittance. Immittance itself is not a physical quantity but simply a term that can be used to refer to either impedance data or admittance data.

In recent years, the measurement of acoustic immittance at the tympanic membrane has become an important component in the basic hearing evaluation. This sensitive and objective diagnostic tool has been used to identify the presence of fluid in the middle ear, to evaluate eustachian tube and facial nerve function, to predict audiometric findings, to determine the nature of hearing loss, and to assist in diagnosing the site of auditory lesion. The application of this technique is considered particularly useful in the assessment of difficult-to-test persons, including very young children.

An example of how this concept may be applied in actual practice is illustrated in Figure 4.13. A pliable probe tip is inserted carefully into the ear canal and an airtight seal obtained so that varying amounts of air pressure can be applied to the ear cavity by pumping air into the ear canal or suctioning it out. A positive amount of air pressure (usually +200 daPa)[a] is then introduced into the airtight ear canal, forcing the tympanic membrane inward. The eardrum is now stiffer than in its natural state because of the positive pressure created in the ear canal. A low-frequency pure tone is then introduced, and a tiny microphone measures the level of the sound reflected from the stiffened eardrum. A low-frequency tone is used because this is the frequency region most affected by changes in stiffness. (See Chapter 2.) Keeping the intensity of the probe tone constant, the pressure is then reduced slowly, causing the tympanic membrane to become more compliant (less stiff). As the tympanic membrane becomes increasingly compliant, more of the acoustic signal will be passed through the middle ear, and the level of the reflected sound in the ear canal will decrease. When the air pressure in the ear canal equals the air pressure in the middle ear, the tympanic membrane will move with the greatest ease. As the pressure is reduced further, the tympanic membrane is pulled in an outward direction, and the eardrum again becomes less mobile. As before, when the eardrum becomes stiffer or less compliant, more low-frequency energy is reflected off the tympanic membrane, and the sound level within the ear canal increases.

An illustration of the basic components found in most immittance instruments is shown in Figure 4.14. The probe tip is sealed in the ear canal, providing

---

[a]daPa represents a measure of air pressure in units of dekapascals. 1 daPa = 10 Pa = 1.02 mm H_2O. Millimeters (mm) H_2O refers to the amount of pressure needed to push a column of water in a special tube to a given height in mm. For measurements of immittance, air pressure is generally expressed relative to ambient air pressure. That is, ambient air pressure is represented as 0 daPa, and a pressure 100 daPa above ambient pressure is represented as +100 daPa.

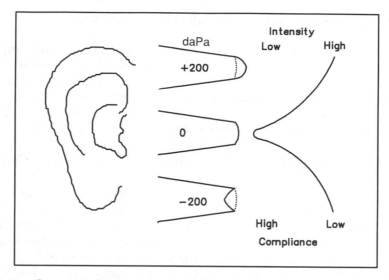

Figure 4.13.   Concepts of immittance applied in practice.

a closed cavity. The probe contains three small ports that are connected to: (*a*) a sound source that generates a low-frequency (usually 220- or 660-Hz) pure tone; (*b*) a microphone to measure the reflected sound wave; and (*c*) an air pump and manometer for varying the air pressure within the ear canal.

Immittance Test Battery

Three basic measurements—tympanometry, static acoustic immittance, and threshold of the acoustic reflex—commonly comprise the acoustic immittance test battery.

Tympanometry

Acoustic immittance at the tympanic membrane of a normal ear changes systematically as air pressure in the external canal is varied above and below

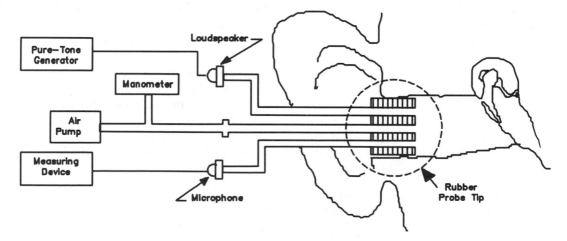

Figure 4.14.   Components of an immittance instrument.

ambient air pressure. This was illustrated previously in Figure 4.13. The normal relationship between air pressure changes and changes in immittance is frequently altered in the presence of middle ear disease. Tympanometry is the measurement of the mobility of the middle ear when air pressure in the external canal is varied from +200 to −400 daPa. Results from tympanometry are then plotted on a graph, with air pressure along the *x* axis and immittance, or *compliance*, along the *y* axis.[b] Figure 4.15 illustrates some of the tympanograms commonly seen in normal and pathologic ears.

Various estimates have been made of the air pressure in the ear canal which results in the least amount of reflected sound energy from normal middle ears. This air pressure is routinely referred to as the peak pressure point. A normal tympanogram for an adult (Fig. 4.15**a**) has a peak pressure point between −100 and +40 daPa, which suggests that the middle ear functions optimally at or near ambient pressure (0 daPa). Tympanograms that peak at a point below the accepted range of normal pressures (Fig. 4.15**b**) suggest malfunction of the middle ear pressure-equalizing system. This malfunction might be due to eustachian tube malfunction, early or resolving serous otitis media, or acute otitis media. (These and other disorders are described in detail in Chapter 5.) Ears that contain fluid behind the eardrum are characterized by a flat tympanogram at a high impedance or low admittance value without a peak pressure point (Fig. 4.15**c**). This implies an excessively stiff system that does not allow for an increase in sound transmission through the middle ear under any pressure state.

The amplitude (height) of the tympanogram also provides information about the compliance or elasticity of the system. A stiff middle ear (as in, for example, ossicular-chain fixation) is represented by a shallow amplitude, suggesting high acoustic impedance or low admittance (Fig. 4.15**d**). Conversely, an ear with abnormally low acoustic impedance or high admittance (as in an interrupted ossicular chain or a hypermobile tympanic membrane) is revealed by a tympanogram having a very high amplitude (Fig. 4.15**e**).

Static Acoustic Immittance

Static acoustic immittance measures the ease of flow of acoustic energy through the middle ear and is usually expressed in "equivalent volume" in cm^3. To obtain this measurement, immittance is first determined under a positive pressure (+200 daPa) artificially induced in the canal. Very little sound is admitted through the middle ear under this extreme positive pressure, with much of the acoustic energy reflected back into the ear canal. Next, a similar determination is made with the eardrum in its most compliant position, thus maximizing transmission through the middle ear cavity. The arithmetic difference between these two immittance values, usually recorded in cubic centimeters (cm^3) of equivalent volume, provides an estimate of immittance at the tympanic membrane. Compliance values less than or equal to 0.25 cm^3 of equivalent volume suggest low acoustic immittance (indicative of stiffening pathologies), and values greater than or equal to 2.0 cm^3 generally indicate abnormally high immittance (suggestive of ossicular discontinuity or healed tympanic membrane perforations).

---

[b]Throughout this text, we have assumed that immittance measurements are made with an impedance meter. With such a device, immittance values are described in arbitrary units, frequently labeled "compliance." These devices do not actually measure compliance.

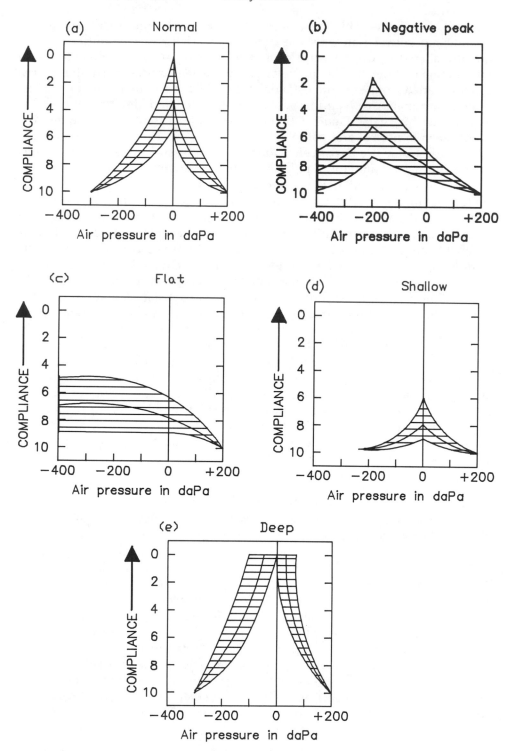

Figure 4.15. Tympanometric configurations seen in normal and pathologic ears.

Acoustic Reflex Threshold

The acoustic reflex threshold is defined as the lowest possible intensity needed to elicit a middle ear muscle contraction. Contraction of the middle ear muscles evoked by intense sound results in a temporary increase in the middle ear impedance. As noted in Chapter 3, the acoustic reflex is a consensual phenomenon; acoustic stimulation to one ear will elicit a muscle contraction and subsequent impedance change in both ears. Traditionally, the acoustic reflex is monitored in the ear canal contralateral to the ear receiving the sound stimulus. An example of how it is measured is shown in Figure 4.16. A headphone is placed on one ear, and the probe assembly is inserted into the contralateral ear. When the signal transduced from the earphone reaches an intensity sufficient to evoke an acoustic reflex, the stiffness of the middle ear is increased in both ears. This results in more sound being reflected from the eardrum, and a subsequent increase in sound pressure is observed on the immittance instrument. In recording the data, it is standard procedure to consider the ear stimulated with the intense sound as the ear under test. Because the ear stimulated is contralateral to the ear in which the reflex is measured, these reflex thresholds are referred to as contralateral reflex thresholds. It is also frequently possible to present the loud reflex-activating stimulus through the probe assembly itself. In this case, the reflex is both activated and measured in the same ear. This is referred to as an ipsilateral acoustic reflex.

In the normal ear, contraction of middle ear muscles occurs with pure tones ranging from 65 to 95 dB HL. A conductive hearing loss, however, tends to either elevate or eliminate the reflex response. When acoustic reflex information is used in conjunction with tympanometry and static acoustic immittance measurements, it serves to substantiate further the existence of a middle ear disorder. With unilateral conductive hearing loss, failure to elicit the reflex is dependent on the size of the air-bone gap and also on the ear in which the probe tip is inserted. If the stimulus is presented to the good ear and the probe tip is placed on the affected side, an air-bone gap of only 10 dB will usually abolish the reflex

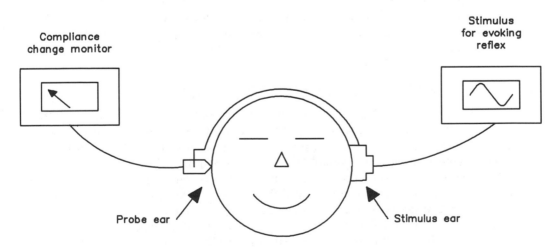

Figure 4.16.   Example of how the acoustic reflex is obtained.

response. If, however, the stimulus is presented to the pathologic ear and the probe is in the normal ear, a gap of 25 dB is needed to abolish or significantly elevate the reflex threshold.

Special Considerations in the Use of Immittance with Young Children

The use of immittance can be most valuable in the assessment of young children, although it does have some diagnostic limitations. Further, although electroacoustic immittance measures are ordinarily simple and quick to obtain, special consideration and skills are required to obtain these measures successfully from young infants.

Although immittance tests may be administered to neonates and young infants with a reasonable amount of success, tympanometry may have limited value with children younger than 7 months of age. Below this age, there is a poor correlation between tympanometry and the actual condition of the middle ear. In very young infants, a normal tympanogram does not necessarily imply that there is a normal middle ear system. However, a flat tympanogram obtained in an infant is highly suggestive of a diseased ear. Consequently, it is still worthwhile to administer immittance tests to this population.

Another limitation of immittance measurements is the difficulty of obtaining measurements on a hyperactive child or a child who is crying, yawning, or continually talking. A young child who exhibits excessive body movement or head turning will make it almost impossible to maintain an airtight seal with the probe tip. Vocalization produces middle ear muscle activity that in turn causes continual alterations in the compliance of the tympanic membrane, making immittance measurements impossible. With difficult-to-test and younger children, specialized techniques are needed to keep the child relatively calm and quiet. For young children, it is always recommended that a second person be involved in the evaluation. While the child is sitting on the parent's lap, one person can place the earphone and insert the probe tip while a second person manipulates the controls of the equipment. With infants below 2 years of age, placing the earphones and headband on the child's head is often distracting. It may be helpful to remove the earphone from the headband, rest the band over the mother's shoulder, and insert the probe tip into the child's ear. It is also helpful to use some distractive techniques that will occupy the child's attention during the test time (Vignette 4.4).

BASIC AUDIOLOGIC TEST BATTERY

In the measurement of auditory function, the most meaningful information can be gleaned only when the entire test battery of pure-tone and speech audiometry together with immittance measurements is used. If just one or two of these procedures are employed, valuable clinical information will be lost, since each of these clinical tools offers a unique and informative set of data. In particular, the reader should keep in mind the differences between pure-tone measures and electroacoustic-immittance measurements. Pure-tone audiometry does not measure the immittance of the middle ear, just as immittance does not measure hearing sensitivity. While an abnormal audiogram strongly suggests the presence of a hearing loss, abnormal immittance does not. Abnormal immittance findings in the absence of significant hearing loss, on the other hand, can be sufficient grounds for medical referral. A test-battery approach is essential. Examples of applications of the test battery are shown in Vignettes 4.5–4.7.

ADDITIONAL SPECIAL TESTS

The basic audiologic test battery determines whether or not the patient has any hearing loss; what effect the hearing loss, if present, has on speech understanding; and whether the nature of the hearing loss is conductive, sensorineural or a combination of the two (mixed). The immittance battery can also evaluate middle ear function regardless of whether a measurable hearing loss is present. Thus, the basic audiologic test battery is able to determine where in the peripheral portion of the auditory system a lesion may be located.

Additional special auditory tests are needed, however, to determine if lesions are present in more centrally located portions of the ascending nervous system, such as the auditory nerve, brainstem, or cortex. A patient with a life-threatening tumor affecting the auditory nerve, for example, will have pure-tone test results consistent with a high-frequency sensorineural hearing loss. Other components of the basic hearing test battery, however, may provide some "warning signs" suggesting that the lesion responsible for the hearing is affecting the auditory nerve. For example, the hearing loss in such cases usually affects the high frequencies and is different in the two ears, often leaving one ear completely unaffected. In addition, speech-recognition scores in the impaired ear are often reduced much more than would be expected on the basis of the pure-tone hearing loss. Finally, acoustic reflex thresholds for the affected ear are typically elevated above the normal range (>100 dB HL). Although these features are typical for many patients with tumors affecting the auditory nerve, there are many cases that manifest only one or two of these features. Patients having inner ear pathology, moreover, may also manifest one or more of these features.

A battery of special auditory tests has been developed to assist in the identification of lesions occurring central to the cochlea or inner ear. These lesions are referred to as retrocochlear lesions. Historically, this test battery was based on a variety of behavioral tests that used pure tones as stimuli. After several years of test development and refinement, most of these tests were still only 60–70% accurate in identifying retrocochlear impairments. Many individuals with cochlear hearing loss were falsely identified as having retrocochlear lesions, and still more retrocochlear lesions were identified as being cochlear in nature.

Today's battery of special auditory tests consists of five basic tests, only one of which involves behavioral measurements in response to pure-tone stimulation (threshold tone decay). The five test procedures measure: (*a*) threshold tone decay; (*b*) performance-intensity functions for speech materials; (*c*) acoustic reflex threshold; (*d*) acoustic reflex decay; and (*e*) auditory brainstem responses (See Chapter 3.). This contemporary test battery is 90–95% accurate in identifying retrocochlear lesions.

Detailed descriptions of these procedures are beyond the scope of this book. It is important to note only that the basic audiologic test battery is limited in its diagnostic usefulness. Additional special auditory tests can be performed in the event that any of the retrocochlear warning signs described above are found after performing the basic tests. Those readers who desire to learn more about the

Vignette 4.4.   Distractive Techniques Used in Evaluating Young Children with Immittance[a]

Flashlight

Direct the light toward the child or shine it on objects or people well within the child's visual field. Constantly change the rate of movement from slow to fast. If habituation occurs, take the child's hand and repeatedly place it over the light source.

Animated Toys

Introduce animated toys only as required at critical times necessary to complete the test. Avoid movement artifacts by keeping the toy well out of the reach of the child.

Cotton Swab

Gently brush the back of the child's hand, arm, or leg in a slow, even motion. Make the distraction visual as well as tactile by making oscillatory or exaggerated movements of the swab.

Pendulum

Using a bright and unusually shaped object, make a pendulum with about an 18-inch string. This technique is highly effective if the examiner swings the pendulum about in various motions within various areas of the infant's vision. Swing the pendulum rather slowly in short excursions, permitting easy visual following. Frequently stop or alter the swinging motion to provide novelty to the pendular action.

Mirror

To an infant less than 1 year of age who is capable of reacting and attending to faces, a large mirror is sometimes irresistible, at least for a period sufficiently long to place a probe tip and to perform the impedance test battery.

Toys That Produce Sounds

Toys or other devices that emit intense sounds should be avoided since they may evoke an acoustic or other reflexive response from the child. Toys that produce softer sounds in no way interfere with the test and can therefore by used effectively, especially if the sound is novel.

Food

Children, like adults, seem to enjoy sweets, and although swallowing and sucking movements are notorious for producing artifacts in the tympanogram and reflex measures, food can still be used as a distractive technique. Flavored gelatin or soft-drink powder in water, honey, or sweetened lemon juice can be dropped into the child's mouth at intervals during the test. Avoid taking measures until the reflexive sucking action has subsided. Administering small amounts of liquid at well-spaced intervals can keep the child occupied for many minutes.

Watch

In front of the child, simply remove one's wristwatch, manipulate or wind it well out of reach of the child or point to it.

---

[a]From Northern JL: Acoustic impedance in the pediatric population. In Bess FH (ed): *Childhood Deafness: Causation, Assessment and Management*. New York, Grune & Stratton, 1977.

Shoe

A simple yet effective technique is to begin lacing and unlacing a child's shoe, either on or off his foot. This should be carefully timed to coincide with the insertion of the test tip into the ear. Move slowly and methodically and do not appear to have any object in mind except to lace and unlace the shoe.

Action Toys

A variety of toys are available that perform repetitive actions, such as a monkey that climbs down a stick pole. Often these are not the best distractive devices because children 1 year and older often wish to handle or manipulate this type of toy.

Wad of Cotton or Tissue

A cotton ball can facilitate effective passive attention by balancing the cotton on the hand, arm, or knee of the child or on the hand of the assistant. It can be squeezed or otherwise manipulated; it can be blown or allowed to fall repeatedly from the hand. A tissue can also be used as a parachute, torn slowly into shapes, rolled into small balls and placed in the child's hand, waved, punctured, and so forth.

Tape

A roll of adhesive or paper surgical tape has been found to be one of the most effective distractive devices available in the clinic. Bits of tape can be torn off or stuck on various parts of the child's or examiner's anatomy. The child can be allowed to pull the tape off, objects can be picked up with the adhesive side of the tape, fingers can be bound together, links can be made with small strips, rings can be formed, fingernails covered, and innumerable other totally nonmeaningful manipulations can be performed. Tape works wonders for the few seconds necessary for obtaining immittance measures.

Lollipop

A lollipop can be utilized when the child is cradled and partially immobilized in the examiner's or parent's arm. The examiner can stroke the child's lips or tongue with the lollipop. Careful spacing of the lollipop sampling permits completion of the entire immittance test pattern.

Miscellaneous Devices

Tongue blades, cotton swabs, colored yarn, or similar devices are all effective as distractive devices. They are best utilized when manipulated or "played with" by the examiner. If the child insists, he can be allowed to manipulate the device. Care must be taken to permit only passive action so as to reduce movement artifact while the test is proceeding.

auditory test battery can consult the Suggested Readings at the end of this chapter.

SUMMARY

We have reviewed the basic components of the test battery used in the measurement of auditory function. This includes the measurement of pure-tone threshold by air and bone conduction, speech audiometry, and immittance measurements. The results from these various approaches, when used as a battery, give the audiologist good insight into the nature and extent of the auditory disorder.

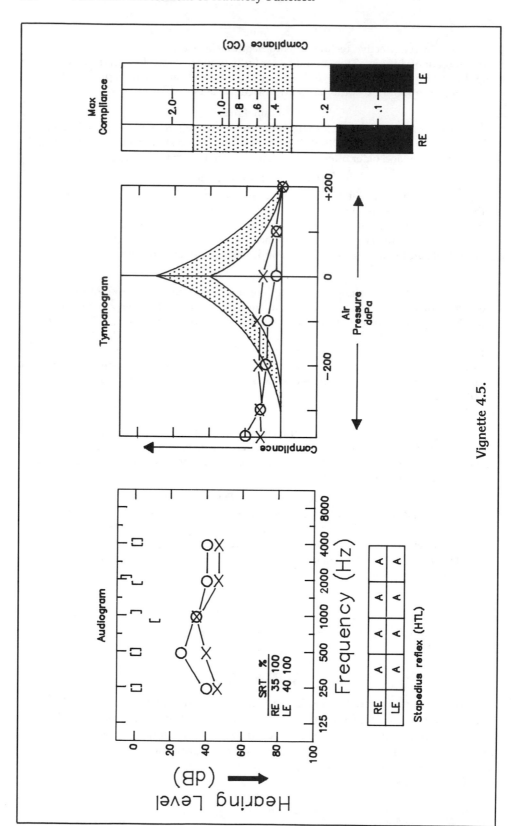

Vignette 4.5.

Vignette 4.5.   A 6-Year-Old Child with Bilateral Otitis Media (see opposing page)

In the accompanying figure, a mild-to-moderate bilateral hearing loss for air conduction is evidenced, whereas bone conduction thresholds are normal in both ears. Such a discrepancy between air conduction and bone conduction thresholds suggests a conductive loss. The speech-recognition thresholds (SRTs) are compatible with the pure-tone data; when the signal is made comfortably loud, suprathreshold speech recognition is excellent in both ears. Good speech recognition is consistent with a middle ear disorder. Immittance confirms the impression of a conductive loss. The shaded areas on the tympanogram and static immittance forms represent normative data. The tympanograms are flat, the static immittance is well below normal, and acoustic reflexes are absent in both ears. This general pattern is consistent with a middle ear complication and highly suggestive of a fluid-filled middle ear, thus requiring a medical referral. If however, there is no evidence of previous middle ear problems and the child has no complaints, a recheck should be recommended in 3 weeks. If the same results are obtained, the child should be referred to the family physician.

Educationally, such a problem can be relatively serious if medical intervention does not result in a speedy return to completely normal hearing levels. Such children are likely to appear listless and inattentive in the classroom, and their performance soon begins to deteriorate. Both the teacher and the parents should receive an explanation of these probable consequences from the audiologist. In counseling the teacher, emphasis should be placed on establishing favorable classroom seating, supplementing auditory input with visual cues, using clear and forceful articulation, and frequent reiteration of assignments. If the condition does not respond readily to medical treatment, consideration of amplification, along with other remedial measures such as speechreading instruction and training in listening skills, should not be ruled out. Above all, the child will need patient understanding during the period when the hearing level is diminished and sometimes fluctuating from one day to the next.

SUPPLEMENT ON "HOW TO MASK"

As mentioned, there are several methods available to mask the nontest ear for measurement of hearing threshold by air and bone conduction. This supplement provides a brief description of a popular method, known as the plateau method (8). This method is very simple and quite popular. Once the audiologist has determined that masking is needed for either air or bone conduction measurements, a low-intensity noise is delivered to the nontest ear. The noise might be a narrow-band noise with frequency content similar to the test tone, or it might be a broad-band noise. Once introduced into the nontest ear, the noise is increased in 5-dB steps until the test tone is no longer heard. Threshold for the tone is then measured again while the noise remains at the same level in the nontest ear. The noise level is increased 5 dB again, and the threshold is then reestablished. During this portion of the plateau method, it is frequently the case that the level of the noise and tone are alternately increased by 5 dB several times. This is because both the tone and the noise are heard in the nontest ear. The tone is heard in that ear because it crosses over through the skull from the

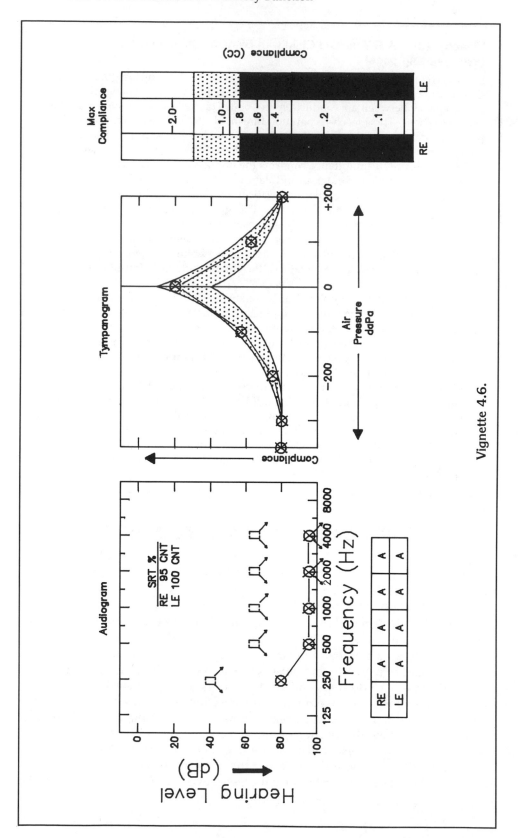

Vignette 4.6.

Vignette 4.6.   An 8-Year-Old Child with a Bilateral Severe-to-Profound Sensorineural Hearing Loss (see opposing page)

The pure-tone results in the accompanying figure display a severe-to-profound sensorineural hearing loss. Bone conduction responses could not be obtained at the maximum output limits of the audiometer. The speech recognition thresholds using selected spondees were compatible with the pure-tone data. Suprathreshold speech-recognition scores could not be obtained because of the severity of the loss. Immittance results on both ears show tympanograms and static immittance values to be within the normal range. Acoustic reflexes are absent in both ears, but these usually cannot be elicited with a hearing loss in excess of 85 dB HL.

These audiologic results confirm the irreversibility of the hearing impairment, which is so severe that the best possible special education opportunities must be made available. Periodic audiologic evaluations are highly important in the optimum educational management of such children. Frequently they may suffer ear infections that further reduce their already greatly depressed level of sensitivity. At such times, the amplification program that has been recommended for them must be modified temporarily while medical treatment is being obtained.

---

test ear while the noise is introduced directly into the nontest ear. Eventually, the noise level will be raised by 5 dB several times with no change in threshold for the pure tone. At this point, the noise has eliminated the participation of the nontest ear in the detection of the tone, and the tone is producing sensation in the test ear. Increasing the noise level under these circumstances causes no shift in hearing threshold for the pure tone because the noise is in the nontest ear and the tone is now being heard in the test ear. The range of noise levels that fail to shift the threshold for the tone is referred to as the plateau. The level of the tone during the plateau represents the true threshold of the test ear at that frequency.

If the noise level in the nontest ear is increased further, the threshold of the pure tone will eventually begin to increase again. This is known as overmasking and occurs when the noise in the nontest ear crosses over through the skull to the test ear and begins to mask the pure tone. During overmasking, the tone and noise will again be alternately increased in 5-dB steps, depending upon the intensity of the noise during the plateau and the output limits of the audiometer. "Minimum masking" occurs at the noise level that first produces the plateau and "maximum masking" occurs at the noise level at the end of the plateau, just prior to overmasking.

Additional details about masking methods are beyond the scope of this introductory text. The reader is referred to Hood (8), Studebaker (9) and Martin (10) for additional details about the plateau method, as well as alternative procedures.

References

1. Egan J: Articulation testing methods. *Laryngoscope* 58:955–991, 1948.
2. Hirsh IJ, Davis H, Silverman SR, Reynolds FG, Eldert E, Benson RW: Development of materials for speech audiometry. *J Speech Hearing Disord* 17:321–337, 1952.
3. Tillman TW, Carhart R: *An Expanded Test for Speech Discrimination Using CNC Monosyllabic Words.* Northwestern University Auditory Test No. 6. Technical Report No. SAM-TR-66-55, USAF School of Aerospace Medicine, Brooks Air Force Base, Texas, 1966.

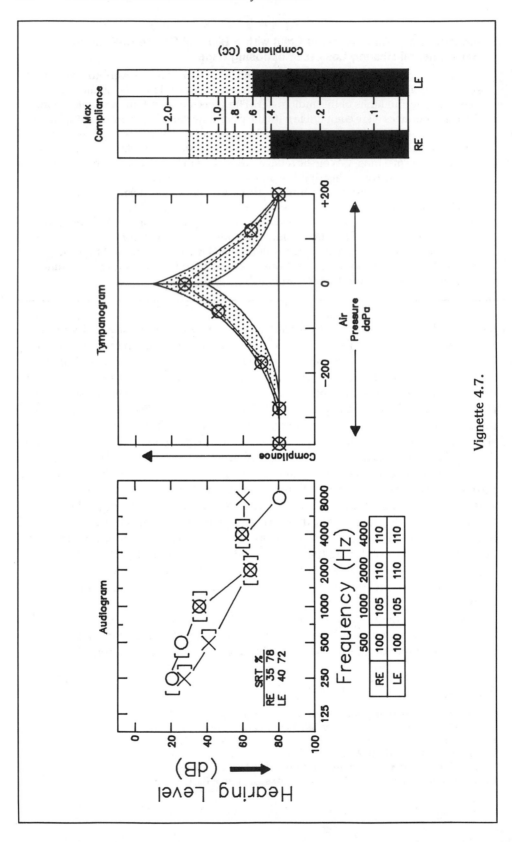

Vignette 4.7.

Vignette 4.7.   Adult with a Bilateral Mild-to-Moderate Sensorineural Hearing Loss (see opposing page)

The pure-tone results accompanying this vignette show a bilateral sloping sensorineural hearing loss in an elderly adult. The speech-recognition thresholds are compatible with the pure-tone data, and suprathreshold speech recognition is only fair to good, even when the signal is made comfortably loud. Immittance results show normal tympanograms and static immittance for both ears, with acoustic reflexes present, but elevated, bilaterally.

Normally, an adult with this battery of results will be either a successful user of individual amplification, a highly competent speechreader, or both. It may still be necessary to provide special assistance in the form of training in auditory and visual communication (speechreading) skills.

---

4.   House AS, Williams CE, Hecker MHL, Kryter KD: Articulation testing methods: consonantal differentiation in a closed-response set. *J Acoust Soc Am* 20:463–474, 1965.

5.   Owens E, Schubert ED: Development of the California consonant test. *J Speech Hear Res* 20:463–474, 1977.

6.   Levitt H, Resnick SB: Speech reception by the hearing impaired: methods of testing and the development of new tests. In Ludvigsen C, Barfod J (eds): *Sensorineural Hearing Impaired and Hearing Aids*. Scand Audiol (Suppl 6):107–130, 1978.

7.   Carhart R: Future horizons in audiological diagnosis. *Ann Otol Rhinol Laryngol* 77:706–716, 1968.

8.   Hood JD: The principles and practice of bone-conduction audiometry: a review of the present position. *Laryngoscope* 70:1211–1228, 1960.

9.   Studebaker GA: Clinical masking in air- and bone-conducted stimuli. *J Speech Hear Disord* 29:23–35, 1964.

10.   Martin FN: Minimum effective masking levels in threshold audiometry. *J Speech Hear Disord* 39:280–285, 1974.

Suggested Readings

American Speech-Language-Hearing Association: Guidelines for audiometric symbols. *ASHA* 16.260–264, 1974.

American Speech-Language-Hearing Association: Guidelines for determining threshold level for speech. *ASHA* 30(3):85–90, 1988.

Bess FH: Clinical assessment of speech recognition. In Konkle DF, Rintelmann WF (eds): *Principles of Speech Audiometry*. Baltimore, University Park Press, 1982.

Bess FH: The minimally hearing impaired child. *Ear Hear*, 6:43–47, 1985.

Bluestone CD, Beery QC, Paradise JL: Audiometry and tympanometry in relation to middle ear effusions in children. *Laryngoscope* 83:594–604, 1963.

Carhart R, Jerger JF: Preferred method for clinical determination of pure-tone thresholds. *J Speech Hear Disord* 24:330–345, 1959.

Diefendorf AO: Pediatric audiology. In Lass NJ, McReynolds LV, Northern JL, Yoder DE (eds): *Handbook of Speech-Language Pathology and Audiology*. Philadelphia, BC Decker, 1988.

Jerger S: Speech audiometry. In Jerger J (ed): *Pediatric Audiology*. San Diego, College Hill Press, 1984.

House AS, Williams CE, Hecker MHL, Kryter KD: Articulation testing methods: consonantal differentiation in a closed-response set. *J Acoust Soc Am* 20:463–474, 1965.

Katz J: *Handbook of Clinical Audiology*, ed 3. Baltimore, Williams & Wilkins, 1985.

Northern JL: Acoustic impedance in the pediatric population. In Bess FH (ed): *Childhood Deafness: Causation, Assessment and Management*. New York, Grune & Stratton, 1977.

Northern JL, Downs MP: *Hearing in Children*, ed 3. Baltimore, Williams & Wilkins, 1984.

Olsen WO, Matkin ND: Speech audiometry. In Rintelmann WF (ed): *Hearing Assessment*. Baltimore, University Park Press, 1979.

Sanders JW: Masking. In Katz J (ed): *Handbook of Clinical Audiology*, ed 2. Baltimore, Williams & Wilkins, 1978, p 124.

Sanders JW: Diagnostic audiology. In Lass NJ, McReynolds NJ, Northern JL, Yoder DE (eds): *Handbook of Speech-Language Pathology and Audiology*. Philadelphia, BC Decker, 1988.

Schwartz D, Josey AF, Bess FH (eds): Proceedings of meeting in honor of Professor Jay Sanders. *Ear Hear* 8:4, 1987.

Shanks JE, Lilly DJ, Margolis RH, Wiley TL, Wilson RH: Tympanometry. *J Speech Hear Disord* 53:354—377, 1988.

Tillman TW, Olsen WO: Speech audiometry. In Jerger J (ed): *Modern Developments in Audiology*. New York, Academic Press, 1973

CHAPTER FIVE

Pathologies of the Auditory System

A variety of disorders, both congenital and acquired, directly affect the auditory system. These disorders can occur at the level of the external ear, the external auditory canal, the tympanic membrane, the middle ear space, the cochlea, the auditory central nervous system, or any combination of these sites. The following review offers a discussion of some of the more commonly seen disorders that can impair the auditory system.

OBJECTIVES

Following completion of this chapter, the reader should be able to:

- Understand the system used to classify auditory disorders.
- Discuss the most common disorders affecting the external ear and middle ear.
- Be familiar with typical disorders affecting the cochlea.
- Identify the most common disorders affecting the auditory central nervous system.
- Develop an appreciation and an understanding of the physical symptoms and audiologic manifestations associated with most of these disorders.

CLASSIFICATION OF AUDITORY DISORDERS

All auditory disorders can be divided into two major classifications: exogenous (outside the genes) and endogenous (within the genes). Exogenous hearing disorders are those caused by inflammatory disease, toxicity, noise, accident, or injury that inflicts damage on any part of the auditory system. Endogenous conditions originate in the genetic characteristics of an individual. An endogenous auditory defect is transmitted from the parents to the child as an inherited trait. However, not all congenital (present at birth) hearing disorders are hereditary, nor are all hereditary disorders congenital. For example, the child whose hearing mechanism is damaged in utero by maternal rubella is born with a hearing loss. This hearing loss is congenital but not hereditary. On the other hand, some hereditary defects of hearing may not manifest themselves until adulthood. A breakdown of the estimated percentage of individuals with exogenous and endogenous types of hearing loss is shown in Figure 5.1.

Genetic Transmission of Hearing Loss

As seen in Figure 5.1, hearing loss due to hereditary factors is thought to make up about 50% of all auditory disorders. It is estimated that there are 150–175 different types of genetic syndromes that include hearing loss as a primary feature. In addition, there are about 16 types of genetic deafness that are known to occur without any other associated anomalies. Whether occurring as one manifestation of a particular syndrome or with no other abnormalities, hereditary hearing loss is usually governed by the Mendelian laws of inheritance. According to these genetic laws, genetic traits may be dominant, recessive, or X linked (sex linked). Genes are located on the chromosomes, and, with the exception of those genes that are located on the sex chromosomes of males, they come in pairs. One member of each gene pair (and the corresponding member of a chromosome pair) is inherited from each parent. Humans have 22 pairs of autosomes, or non-sex-determining chromosomes, and one pair of sex-determining chromosomes. The sex chromosome pair for females consists of two X chromosomes, and for males, one X and one Y chromosome. In the process of human reproduction, each egg and each sperm cell carries one half the number of chromosomes of each parent. When the egg is fertilized, the full complement of chromosomes is restored, so that half of a child's genes are from the mother and half from the father.

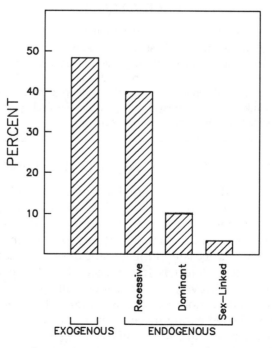

Figure 5.1. Percentage of individuals that exhibit exogenous and endogenous types of hearing loss.

Autosomal Dominant Inheritance

In autosomal dominant inheritance, the trait is carried from one generation to another. The term "autosomal" implies that the abnormal gene is not located on one of the two sex chromosomes. Typically, one parent exhibits the inherited trait, which may be transmitted to 50% of the offspring. This does not mean that half the children in a given family will necessarily be affected. Statistically, there is a 50% chance that any given child, whether male or female, will be affected (Vignette 5.1). Autosomal dominant inheritance is believed to account for about 20% of cases of genetically caused deafness (endogenous). Because of the interaction of a number of genes, some traits may manifest themselves only partially; for example, only a very mild hearing loss may be observed despite a genetic structure indicating profound hearing loss.

Autosomal Recessive Inheritance

In contrast to autosomal dominant inheritance, both parents of a child with hearing loss of the autosomal recessive type are clinically normal. Appearance of the trait in the offspring requires that an individual possess two similar abnormal genes, one from each parent. The parents themselves are heterozygous carriers of a single abnormal recessive gene. This means that each carries two different genes, one normal and one abnormal with respect to a particular gene pair. Offspring carrying two of either the normal or the abnormal type of gene are termed homozygotes. Offspring may also be heterozygotes like their parents, carrying one of each gene type. If no abnormal gene is transmitted, the offspring is normal for that trait. If there is one abnormal gene, the child becomes a carrier for the trait. Finally, if two abnormal genes, one from each parent, are transmitted, the offspring is affected and becomes a homozygous carrier. The probability that heterozygote parents will bear an affected, homozygous child is 25% in each pregnancy on the basis that each child would inherit the abnormal gene from both the father (50% chance) and the mother (50% chance). Since the laws of probability permit this type of hearing loss to be transmitted without manifestation through several generations, the detection of the true origin is often quite difficult. Recessive genes account for the majority of cases of genetic hearing loss and can account for as much as 80% of childhood deafness.

X-Linked Inheritance

In the X-linked type of deafness, affected males are linked together through carrier females. In this pattern, inherited traits are determined by genes located on the X chromosome. As noted earlier, normal females have two X chromosomes, while males possess one X and one Y chromosome. Sons receive their Y chromosomes from their fathers; their X chromosomes are inherited from their mothers. Daughters, on the other hand, receive one X chromosome from their fathers and the other from their mothers. In an X-linked trait, a carrier female has a 50% probability that each of her sons will be affected and a 50% probability that each of her daughters could be carriers. All the daughters of an affected male would be carriers, but there is never a father-to-son transmission of the trait itself. About 2–3% of deafness occurs as a result of X-linked inheritance.

Vignette 5.1. Illustration of Mendelian Laws

For this demonstration, you will need two paper cups and five poker chips or checkers: three of one color and two of another. For the first illustration, select one chip of one color and three of the other color. We will assume that you have one black chip and three white ones. Divide the four chips into two pairs, each pair representing a parent. The black chip represents a dominant gene for deafness. Whenever it is paired with another black chip or a white chip, it dominates the trait for hearing, resulting in deafness in the person with the gene. In this example, we have one deaf parent (one black chip, one white chip) and one normal-hearing parent (two white chips).

Each parent contributes one gene for hearing status to each offspring. When the deaf parent contributes the gene for deafness (black chip), the offspring will always be deaf. This is because the normal-hearing parent has only recessive genes for normal hearing (white chips) to contribute to the offspring. Separate the black chip from the deaf parent and slide it toward you. Slide each of the white chips from the other parent toward you, one at a time. For both of these possible offspring, the child will be deaf (a black chip paired with a white one). Now return the chips to the parents and slide the white chip from the deaf parent close to you. Slide each of the white chips from the normal parent closer to you, one after the other. Notice that when the deaf parent contributes a gene for normal hearing (white chip) parent, the offspring will have normal hearing. This is true for pairings of each gene from the normal-hearing parent. For these two possible gene pairings, the offspring would have normal hearing.

In toto, there were four possible gene pairings for the offspring. Of these, two were predicted to be deaf and two were predicted to be normal. In this illustration of autosomal dominant deafness, the odds are that 50%, or one-half, of the offspring from these two parents will be deaf.

Now, remove one of the white chips and replace it with a black one. Form two pairs of chips in front of you, each having one black and one white chip. In this case, the black chip represents the gene for deafness again, but it is recessive. That is, the gene for normal hearing (white chip) is dominant. There will again be four possible pairings of the chips in the offspring, one from each parent. Examine the various combinations of genes by first sliding one chip closer to you from the parent on the left. Examine two possible pairings for each gene from the parent on the right. Now repeat this process by sliding the other chip from the parent on the left closer to you. When you have finished, you should have observed the following four pairs of chips for the offspring (black-white, black-black, white-black, white-white). In this case of autosomal recessive deafness, only one of the possible combinations would produce a deaf offspring (black-black). The probability of a deaf child is one in four, or 25%. Two of the three normal-hearing offspring, however, will carry a gene for deafness (black-white chip pairs). These offspring are referred to as "carriers" of the trait.

It is sometimes difficult to understand that the Mendelian laws of hearing are only probabilities. In the case of autosomal recessive deafness, for example, one might think that if the parents had four offspring, they would have one deaf child. That is only the probability. They could very well have four normal-hearing children or four deaf children. To see how this occurs, place one black and one white chip in each of the two paper cups. Shake up the left cup and draw a chip. Repeat the process with the right cup. Examine the two chips (genes) selected, one from each cup (parent). Record the outcome (deaf or normal hearing) and replace chips in the cups. Do this 20 times, representing five families of four offspring each. When you're finished, you will likely find some families of four that had two, three, or four deaf offspring. If you did this an *infinite* number of times, however, 25% of the offspring would be deaf, as predicted by Mendelian laws for autosomal recessive deafness.

Site of Lesion

Also important in the classification of an auditory disorder is the location of the lesion. We have already learned that lesions occurring in the outer or middle ear cause conductive hearing loss that is frequently amenable to medical treatment. If damage occurs to the nerve endings or to the hair cells in the inner ear, the hearing loss is sensorineural. Hearing losses resulting from damage to the auditory nerve after it leaves the cochlea are sometimes designated neural. When damage occurs to the nerve pathways within the auditory central nervous system (Chapter 3), the resulting condition is often known as central auditory impairment.

One other variable that can be used in the classification of auditory disorders, but is not in need of detailed explanation here, is time of onset. Typically, the hearing loss is described, in part, with consideration of when the impairment was thought to occur (i.e., prior to delivery or after birth). Time of onset will be discussed in more detail later in this chapter.

DISORDERS OF THE OUTER EAR AND MIDDLE EAR

Conductive hearing losses occur when there exists a complication somewhere between the outer ear and the middle ear. A person with a conductive hearing loss exhibits normal threshold sensitivity by bone conduction measurements and decreased threshold values via air conduction. In the previous chapter, this was referred to as an air-bone gap.

A variety of disorders can produce a conductive hearing loss. All of them result in the alteration of the mechanics of the external ear or the middle ear system. Some of these mechanical changes might include blockage of the external or middle ear, increasing the stiffness of the tympanic membrane or middle ear system, or increasing the mass of the middle ear. These alterations in the mechanics of the outer and middle ear produce varying degrees and configurations of hearing loss. Recall from Chapter 2 that increasing the stiffness of a mechanical system has its greatest effect at low frequencies. Similarly, changing the mass of a mechanical system primarily affects the high frequencies. The specific configuration of the audiogram will depend on the specific mechanical alterations produced by the disorder. Although the conductive loss might make it difficult to hear conversational speech, the ability to understand spoken messages is usually not impaired when speech is presented at comfortably loud levels.

Outer Ear Disorders

Deformities of the Pinna (Auricle) and External Ear Canal

A wide variety of external ear malformations or anomalies can take place, with most due to an inherited trait. Such anomalies of the external ear can occur in isolation or as part of an anomaly complex that produces a variety of other alterations to the skull and face (called craniofacial defects). Pinna deformity can range from very mild malformations, which are difficult for the lay person to identify, to the more severe forms of the condition, such as total absence of the pinna or complete closure of the ear canal.

The most severe form of pinna deformity is called *microtia,* a term that implies a very small and deformed pinna. Microtia is often associated with *atresia,* a term used to denote the absence or closure of the external auditory meatus. Importantly, atresia can also occur without significant pinna abnormalities or as part of a constellation of other craniofacial defects. Examples of the variations in pinna deformities are shown in Figure 5.2.

Microtia and atresia are bilateral in 15–20% of cases, are known to affect the right ear more frequently than the left, and are slightly more prevalent in males.

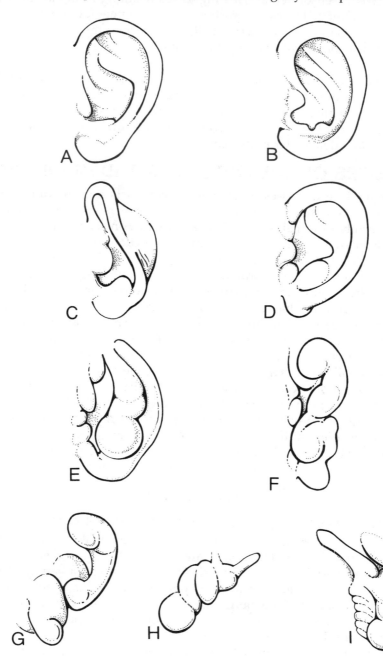

Figure 5.2.   Examples of variations in pinna deformities.

The severity of the pinna deformity will sometimes offer an indication of the corresponding status of the middle ear space. A patient with microtia, for example, can also exhibit malformations of the middle ear ranging from minor deformities of the ossicles to a total absence of the middle ear cavity. Generally speaking, the more severe the deformation of the outer ear, the greater the conductive hearing loss. An example of a conductive hearing loss seen in a severe case of microtia is shown in Figure 5.3.

External Otitis

A number of diseases can cause acute external otitis, which originates from viruses or bacteria. One of these diseases, referred to as herpes simplex, invades the pinna or ear canal. The disease resembles the herpes seen on the face or other parts of the body. Another inflammatory disease is viral bullous myringitis, a complication that involves the outer layer of the tympanic membrane and then spreads laterally to the external canal. In rare instances, these diseases can produce severe swelling of the canal and subsequent hearing loss.

Collapsed Canal

An occasional clinical finding is the collapse of an ear canal brought about by the pressure that results from earphone placement. The pressure of the earphones against the side of the head moves the pinna forward and thus causes the soft cartilaginous part of the ear canal to close. This condition is thought to

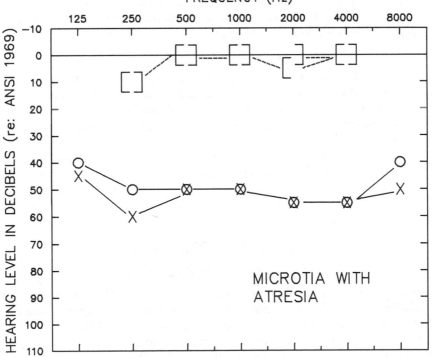

Figure 5.3.   Audiometric example of hearing loss seen in a severe case of bilateral microtia with atresia.

occur in about 3% of a clinical caseload and affects both children and adults. There is a tendency, however, for this condition to occur more frequently in adults, especially in the elderly population. Importantly, the collapsed canal has also been reported to occur in neonates. A collapse of the ear canal can produce a conductive hearing impairment on the order of 15–30 dB HL, with the greatest loss occurring at 2000 Hz. The use of insert earphones, described in Chapter 4, eliminates the problem of collapsing ear canals.

Cerumen and Foreign Bodies

In some individuals, the ear canal generates excessive amounts of cerumen (earwax). If not removed on a periodic basis, this can accumulate and block the transmission of sound to the middle ear. The ear canal is also sufficiently large to accept foreign objects such as matches, paper clips, and pencil tips. Portions of these objects inserted by either children or adults can be lost in the ear canal and remain there for many years. This can result in mild forms of conductive hearing loss. Those audiologists who plan to specialize in the pediatric population should recognize that children have been known to insert seeds or beans into the ear canal. The ear canal is warm and moist and provides an excellent growing environment! When the seed or bean expands, the child experiences pain and loss of hearing.

Finally, sharp objects inserted into the ear canal have the potential for piercing or tearing the tympanic membrane. Such trauma can also cause disruption of the ossicular chain. Self-induced perforations of the tympanic membrane and/or separation of the ossicles can result in a mild-to-moderate conductive hearing loss. The audiologist should make a practice of inspecting the ear canal with an otoscope prior to conducting an audiologic examination.

Cysts and Tumors

The external ear and ear canal can serve as a site for both cysts and tumors. A cyst is a closed cavity or sac that lies underneath the skin and is often filled with a liquid or semisolid material. A cyst is primarily of cosmetic importance unless it becomes infected. It is possible for the swelling resulting from infection to cause hearing loss.

Tumors, both benign and malignant, can arise from the pinna or ear canal. Benign tumors can have a vascular origin or simply represent an outgrowth of bone. Malignancies more frequently arise from the pinna but can, in rare circumstances, arise in the ear canal. Occasionally, these lesions become quite large and close off the ear canal.

Middle Ear Disorders

The Problem of Otitis Media

An important middle ear disorder frequently seen by the audiologist is otitis media—a disorder that constitutes one of the most common diseases in childhood. Otitis media refers to inflammation of the middle ear cavity. It is considered an important economic and health problem because of its prevalence, the cost of its treatment, the potential for secondary medical complications, and the possibility of long-term nonmedical consequences. The clinical audiologist must be familiar with this middle ear disorder and have a grasp of such important topics as the classification of otitis media, its natural history and epidemiology, its cause, its management, and its potential complications.

Classification of Otitis Media

Otitis media is often classified on the basis of a temporal sequence. That is, the disease is categorized according to the duration of the disease process. For example, acute otitis media (AOM) typically will run its full course within a 3-week period. The disease begins with a rapid onset, persists for a week to 10 days, and then exhibits rapid resolution. Some of the more common symptoms associated with AOM include a bulging, reddened tympanic membrane, pain, and upper respiratory infection. If the disease has a slow onset and persists for a period of 3 months or more, it is referred to as chronic otitis media (COM). Symptoms associated with COM include a large central perforation in the eardrum and discharge of fluid through the perforation. Subacute otitis media refers to a disease that has persisted beyond the acute stage but has not yet become chronic.

Otitis media is also classified according to the type of fluid that is observed by the physician in the middle ear cavity. If the fluid is purulent or suppurative, like the fluid found most often in AOM, it will contain white blood cells, some cellular debris, and many bacteria. AOM is sometimes referred to as acute suppurative otitis media or acute purulent otitis media. A fluid that is free of cellular debris and bacteria is described as *serous*, and the term *serous otitis media* is used to describe this condition. Sometimes the fluid is mucoid because it has been secreted from the mucosal lining of the middle ear. This fluid is thick in substance and contains white blood cells, few bacteria, and some cellular debris. When mucoid fluid is present, the disease may be referred to as mucoid otitis media, or secretory otitis media. A summary of the most commonly employed descriptions of otitis media and their associated synonyms is shown in Table 5.1. In addition, Figure 5.40 illustrates a normal tympanic membrane along with several pathologic conditions including serous otitis media, otitis media with bubbles in the fluid, and acute otitis media.

Natural History and Epidemiology of Otitis Media

To understand fully the nature of otitis media, one must develop an appreciation for the natural history and epidemiology of the disease. *Natural history* and *epidemiology* are terms used to denote the study of the relationships of various

Table 5.1.
Clinical Classification of Otitis Media and Commonly Used Synonyms

Classification	Synonyms
Otitis media without effusion	Myringitis
Acute otitis media	Suppurative OM,[a] purulent OM, bacterial OM
Otitis media with effusion	Secretory OM, nonsuppurative OM, serous OM, mucoid OM
Chronic otitis media	Suppurative OM, purulent OM

[a]OM, otitis media.

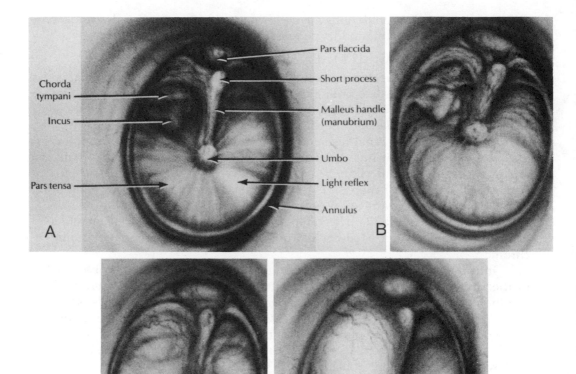

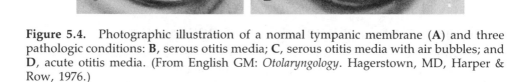

Figure 5.4. Photographic illustration of a normal tympanic membrane (**A**) and three pathologic conditions: **B**, serous otitis media; **C**, serous otitis media with air bubbles; and **D**, acute otitis media. (From English GM: *Otolaryngology.* Hagerstown, MD, Harper & Row, 1976.)

factors that determine the natural frequency and distribution of a disease. It has already been stated that otitis media with effusion is one of the most prevalent diseases in childhood. Depending on the study reviewed, 76–95% of all children have at least one episode of otitis media by 6 years of age. In addition, it is found that the prevalence of the disease peaks during the early years of life. The prevalence of otitis media is typically greatest during the first 2 years of life and then decreases with increasing age. Importantly, there appears to be a relationship between the age of onset and the probability of repeated episodes. Children who appear to be prone to middle ear disease and experience five to six bouts within the first several years of life have usually experienced their first episode of the disease during the first 18 months of life. Seldom does a child become otitis prone if the first episode occurred after 18 months of age.

Otitis media varies slightly with gender, with more cases seen in males than in females. There is seasonal variation in otitis media, with higher occurrence during winter and spring. Some groups are more at risk for middle ear disease than others. Some of the groups considered more at risk for otitis media include children with cleft palate and other craniofacial disorders, those with Down syndrome, and those with learning disabilities. Children who reside in the inner city and children who attend day-care centers are also prone to suffer from middle ear disease, as are American Indians.

Cause of Otitis Media

It is commonly believed that otitis media develops because of eustachian tube obstruction. As mentioned in Chapter 3, the eustachian tube is important to a healthy middle ear because it provides for pressure equalization and fluid drainage. If the pressure-equalization system is obstructed, a negative pressure can develop in the middle ear cavity. The negative pressure literally sucks the fluid from the membranous lining of the middle ear canal. The fluid that has accumulated from the mucosal lining of the middle ear has no place to escape because the eustachian tube is blocked. A representation of this general process is shown in Vignette 5.2. There are a number of possible factors that may produce eustachian tube obstruction, including large adenoid tissue in the nasopharyngeal area and inflammation of the mucous lining of the tube.

Nonmedical Complications Associated with Otitis Media

Hearing loss is considered the most common complication of otitis media. Although the nature of the loss is usually conductive, sensorineural involvement can also occur. In general, the prevalence rate is dependent on the criteria used to define hearing loss. Unfortunately, prevalence data are difficult to determine because of the lack of well-controlled studies in this area. Too often, there is limited information with regard to testing conditions, calibration of equipment, type of threshold procedure employed, definition of hearing loss, and diagnosis of the disease.

An audiometric profile typical of individuals having otitis media with effusion is shown in Figure 5.5. It is seen that the hearing loss for air conduction is fairly flat. The average amount of air conduction loss through the speech frequency range (500–2000 Hz) is 25 dB HL. The bone conduction loss averages 3 dB HL through the speech frequencies, producing a mean air-bone gap of roughly 22 dB.

The degree of hearing loss ranges from normal sensitivity to hearing losses as great as 50 dB HL. A distribution of the expected hearing loss subsequent to otitis media with effusion is shown in Figure 5.6. These data illustrate the number of ears falling within various hearing loss categories. Within the speech frequency range, fewer than 50 ears (7.7%) showed an average loss of 10 dB HL or less, and only five ears showed losses of 50 dB HL or more. The vast majority of ears exhibited losses between 16 and 40 dB HL, with 21–30 dB HL representing the most common hearing loss category.

Although otitis media is usually manifested as a conductive hearing loss, sensorineural hearing loss may be associated with the more severe forms of COM. It is believed that toxic products from the fluid can pass through the round window and damage the cochlea. The damage to the inner ear produces high-

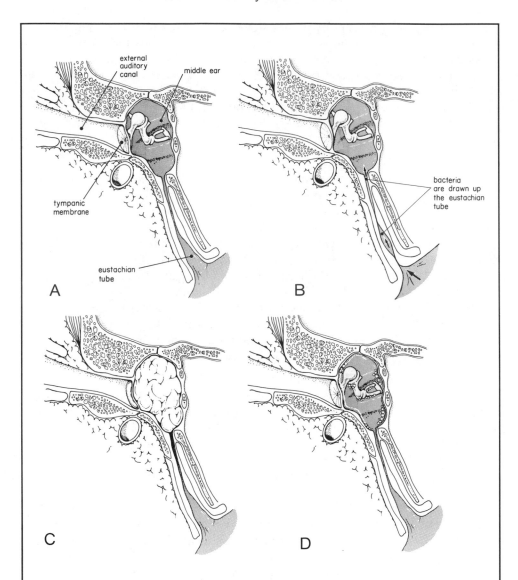

Vignette 5.2.   Development of Acute Otitis Media (AOM)

The drawings that accompany this vignette illustrate the general pattern of events that can occur in AOM. Panel **A** shows the landmarks of a normal middle ear system. Note the translucency and concavity of the tympanic membrane. Note also the appearance of the eustachian tube, especially at the opening in the nasopharyngeal area. In panel **B** it is seen that the pharyngeal end of the eustachian tube has been closed off by swelling due to pharyngeal infection or possibly an allergy. More specifically, the upper respiratory infection produces a congestion of the mucosa in the nasopharyngeal area, the eustachian tube, and the middle ear. The congestion of the mucosa of the tube produces an obstruction that prevents ventilation of the middle ear space. It is also seen that the tympanic membrane is retracted inward because of negative pressure due to absorption from the middle ear. Finally, bacteria from the oral pharyngeal area are drawn up the eustachian tube to the middle ear space. The panel **C** illustrates a full-blown condition of AOM. Fluid secretions from the goblet cells of the mucosa lining of the middle ear are now trapped and have no way to leave the middle ear cavity. The bacteria drawn from the eustachian tube proliferate in the secretions, forming a viscous pus. Observe also that the tympanic membrane is no longer retracted but is bulging.

Panel **D** shows a condition that may well result following antimicrobial treatment. The bacteria have been killed by the antibiotics, and a thin or mucoid-type fluid remains. Other possible outcomes following medical treatment might be the return to a completely normal middle ear, as in **A**, or a condition as in **B**.

The onset of otitis media with effusion, although asymptomatic, would follow a similar pattern of events. Recurrent episodes of AOM or middle ear disease with effusion are probably due to abnormal anatomy or physiology of the eustachian tube.

---

frequency sensorineural hearing loss. The longer the fluid remains in the middle ear, the greater the sensorineural involvement.

Another complication that may result from longstanding middle ear disease with effusion is difficulty in psychoeducational and/or communicative skills. It is widely suspected that otitis-prone children are more susceptible to delays in speech, language, and cognitive development, and in education. The research done in this area, however, has been severely criticized and a cause-effect relationship cannot be assumed at the present time.

Medical Complications Associated with Otitis Media

There are a number of medical complications associated with otitis media. The most common medical complications are COM with associated cholesteatoma, perforations or retraction pockets of the tympanic membrane, tympanosclerosis, adhesive otitis media, and facial paralysis.

COM and Associated Cholesteatoma.   Cholesteatoma refers to the accumulation of cellular debris developed from perforations of the tympanic membrane. Sometimes this pseudotumor becomes infected and causes some erosion of the ossicles. There is no typical audiometric configuration associated with cholesteatomas, and the loss may vary from 15 to 55 dB HL.

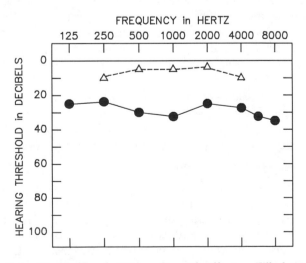

Figure 5.5.   Audiometric profile of otitis media with effusion. Filled circles represent air conduction thresholds; open triangles represent bone conduction thresholds.

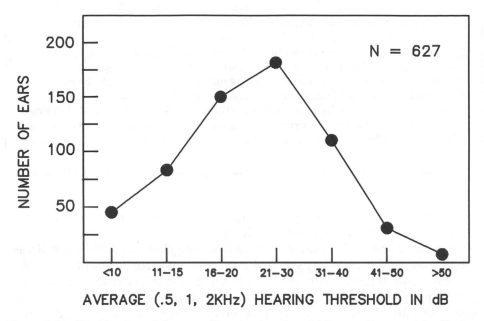

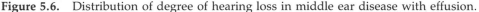

Figure 5.6.   Distribution of degree of hearing loss in middle ear disease with effusion.

Perforation of the Tympanic Membrane.   Spontaneous perforations usually occur subsequent to acute infections but may also be associated with COM. Perforations of the tympanic membrane produce hearing deficits in the mild-to-moderate category, provided there are no ossicular defects. The hearing loss is a result of reduction in the areal ratio between the tympanic membrane and oval window and the direct coupling of sound waves to the round window. (See Chapter 3 for a discussion of these mechanisms.) Figure 5.7 illustrates several different perforations of the tympanic membrane.

Tympanosclerosis.   Tympanosclerosis is characterized by white shale-like plaques on the tympanic membrane and deposits on the ossicles. It occurs most often following COM, which, when resolved, leaves a residual material. The shale-like plaques create a stiffening effect on the tympanic membrane and the ossicular chain, producing conductive hearing loss in the low frequencies.

Adhesive Otitis Media.   Adhesive otitis media is a thickening of the mucous membrane lining the middle ear cavity. It can cause fixation of the ossicles and subsequent hearing loss.

Facial Paralysis.   Facial paralysis may occur in the course of acute or chronic otitis media. The facial nerve passes through the middle ear area in a bony tube called the fallopian canal. It is possible for the fallopian canal to become eroded and expose the facial nerve to the toxic effects of the infection.

Management of Otitis Media

The most common means of treating AOM is by the routine administration of antimicrobial agents. These antibiotics are designed to combat the various pathogens thought to exist within the middle ear fluid. The drug ampicillin appears to be the most effective and most frequently administered drug in the management of AOM. Importantly, even when appropriate antimicrobial agents

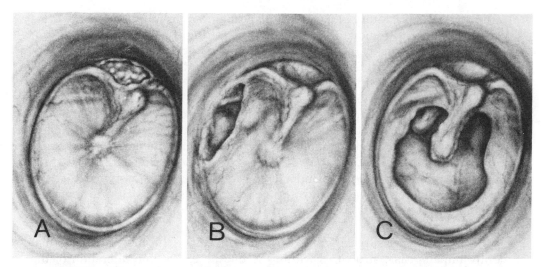

Figure 5.7.   Photographic illustrations of perforations in three different tympanic membranes (From English GM: *Otolaryngology*. Hagerstown, MD, Harper & Row, 1976.)

have been prescribed and the fluid is sterilized, the effusion may persist for 2 weeks to 3 months. Antihistamines and decongestants have also been used in the treatment of middle ear disease. This form of treatment, however, has recently been shown to be ineffective.

A common surgical approach to the management of both suppurative and nonsuppurative otitis media is a myringotomy. Myringotomy is a surgical procedure that involves making an incision in one of the inferior quadrants of the tympanic membrane, as shown in Figure 5.8. In the acute forms of the disease, a myringotomy is performed when there is severe pain or toxicity, high fever, failure to respond to antimicrobial therapy, or some serious secondary medical

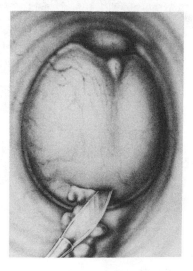

Figure 5.8.   Illustration of myringotomy. Note the bulging appearance of the tympanic membrane (From English GM: *Otolaryngology*. Hagerstown, MD, Harper & Row, 1976.)

complication. In secretory otitis media, a myringotomy is more commonly done usually in order to remove fluid and restore hearing sensitivity. The eardrum incision can heal quickly, however, and the fluid reappears. To avoid this possibility and to ensure sustained middle ear aeration, ventilating tubes or grommets are often inserted into the eardrum (Fig. 5.9).

Tonsillectomy and adenoidectomy are also considered as a management approach to otitis media. While tonsillectomy does not seem to be an effective treatment protocol, adenoidectomy is a common surgical procedure for the management of otitis media. In general, this approach is undertaken when a patient does not respond to medical therapy, large adenoids are present, and there is no evidence of nasal allergy. Under these conditions, it is assumed that the eustachian tube blockage causing the middle ear disease is due to enlarged adenoids. The adenoids are removed to free the eustachian tube from the blockage.

A more radical surgical approach is required if a chronic disease permanently impairs basic structures within the middle ear. When alteration of the middle ear structures is required, a surgical technique known as tympanoplasty is performed.

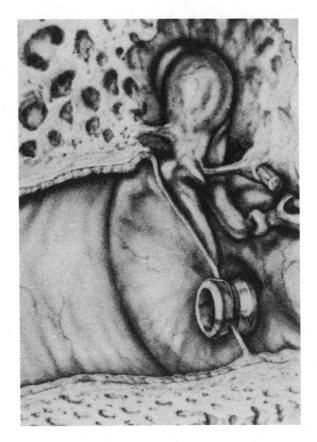

Figure 5.9. Photographic illustration of ventilating tubes or grommets (From English GM: *Otolaryngology*. Hagerstown, MD, Harper & Row, 1976).

Otosclerosis

Otosclerosis, sometimes referred to as otospongiosis, is a common cause of conductive hearing loss and is reported to affect 5–10% of the Caucasian population. Otosclerosis means "hardening of the ear" and is manifested by a buildup of spongifying bone on the osseous labyrinth, usually in the area of the oval window. The buildup of bone around the oval window immobilizes the footplate of the stapes and interferes with sound transmission to the inner ear. Although the focus of the lesion is usually limited to the region of the oval window, the growth of spongy bone can also invade the walls of the cochlea. When the cochlea becomes involved, sensorineural hearing loss may ensue, producing a condition called cochlear otosclerosis.

The disease is about 2.5 times as common in women as in men and may be exacerbated during pregnancy. The disease occurs less frequently in blacks and Orientals and usually has its onset when the individuals are in their 20s, 30s, or 40s. Finally, bilateral otosclerosis is much more common than unilateral disease, although the latter will be seen in 10–15% of the cases.

The cause of otosclerosis is not clearly understood. Most would agree that the disease has a genetic predisposition, since about 50% of affected patients report a similar condition in other family members. The mode of transmission is thought to be autosomal dominant with variable expressivity.

Audiologic Manifestations of Otosclerosis

A progressive conductive hearing loss is the primary result of otosclerosis. The affected patient will typically exhibit an audiometric configuration similar to that shown in Figure 5.10. This figure depicts the air and bone conduction thresholds of a 35-year-old female patient with surgically confirmed otosclerosis. The hearing loss has progressed somewhat gradually for several years, beginning at the age of 25 years. Notice the moderate hearing thresholds for air conduction with greater loss in the low-frequency region, and the relatively normal bone conduction thresholds. An exception to the latter is the slight reduction of bone conduction hearing at 2000 Hz. The bone conduction loss at 2000 Hz is characteristic of otosclerosis and is referred to as the "Carhart notch" because Carhart was the first to report this notching phenomenon. Immittance measurements in otosclerotic cases are also uniquely characteristic and typically manifest absent acoustic reflexes, abnormally low compliance values, and a shallow tympanogram. An audiometric example of a patient with both stapedial and cochlear involvement from otosclerosis is shown in Figure 5.11. Note that a mixed hearing loss is present, representing a conductive component due to stapes fixation and a sensorineural component due to the spread of the spongy bone to the cochlea.

Management of Otosclerosis

The most common approach to the management of otosclerosis is surgery of the stapes. The ideal candidates for stapes surgery are those with relatively normal bone conduction thresholds (0–20 dB HL, 500–2000 Hz) and air conduction values in the 35- to 65-dB HL range (500–2000 Hz). Surgical candidates usually exhibit an air-bone gap of at least 15 dB and have speech-recognition scores of 60% or better.

One surgical approach to otosclerosis is a stapes mobilization, which is

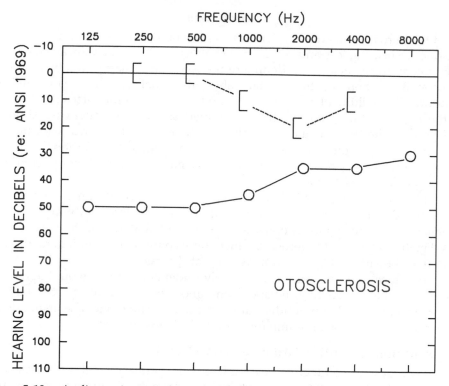

Figure 5.10.   Audiometric example of otosclerosis.

simply a loosening of the stapes with a chisel-like instrument. A limitation of this technique is that in many cases the fixation of the stapes and subsequent conductive hearing loss can recur. An alternative and more accepted approach is the stapedectomy. A stapedectomy involves removal of the fixed stapes footplate and all or a portion of the stapedial arch and substitution of a prosthetic device for the stapes. In cases of complete stapedectomy and the incorporation of a prosthetic device, the oval window is sealed with a graft or an absorptive sponge. Surgery usually results in complete or nearly complete restoration of hearing. Examples of two surgical procedures are shown in Figure 5.12.

Other Ossicular Disorders

The ossicles other than the stapes can also be partially or completely fixed. The ossicles can also be pulled apart, or disarticulated, producing a variety of different conductive hearing losses. For example, the malleus and the incus can become fixated, or there can be fixation of the malleus alone or the incus alone without any involvement of the stapes. These conditions are sometimes referred to as "pseudo-otosclerosis," and the audiologic manifestations often mock what we would expect to find in otosclerosis.

In contrast to fixation, it is possible to have discontinuity, or disarticulation, of the ossicles, again producing a significant conductive hearing loss. A discontinuity of the ossicles can be caused by a degenerative process or by some traumatic experience. For example, the introduction of a sharp object into the ear canal could pierce the tympanic membrane and cause a dislocation of the ossicles. A

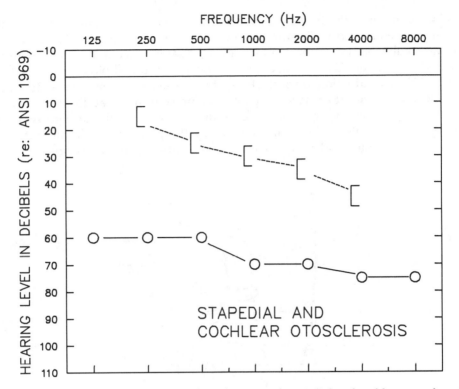

Figure 5.11. Audiometric example of combination of stapedial and cochlear otosclerosis.

similar effect can result from a skull fracture where the impact to the head produces a dislodging of the ossicular chain. In addition, it is possible to note degeneration of the ossicles when a disease process (particularly a cholesteatoma) is present. Under these conditions, the individual will exhibit a substantial conductive hearing loss in the neighborhood of 50–60 dB.

COCHLEAR AND RETROCOCHLEAR PATHOLOGY

Millions of Americans have sensorineural hearing loss as a consequence of cochlear pathology. For children, conductive hearing loss produced by middle ear pathology, as reviewed in the previous portion of this chapter, is probably the most common type of hearing loss. For adults, however, sensorineural hearing loss resulting from underlying cochlear pathology is probably the most common type of hearing impairment. Recall from the previous sections of this chapter that conductive hearing loss was usually medically treatable, either through surgery, medication, or a combination of the two. With sensorineural hearing loss, however, this is usually not the case. The hearing loss is typically permanent. For those individuals with significant sensorineural hearing loss, the usual course of action is to seek assistance from amplification, often a personal wearable hearing aid. Hearing aids and other types of amplification for the hearing impaired are described in detail in Chapter 7.

The description of the hearing loss produced by cochlear pathology as "sensorineural" seems particularly appropriate. Recall that a sensorineural hearing loss is one in which the threshold by bone conduction is the same as that by air conduction (within 5 dB). The threshold when the inner ear is stimulated directly through skull vibration (bone conduction) is the same as when the entire peripheral auditory system is stimulated (air conduction). If thresholds for air conduction and bone conduction are both elevated to the same degree, then all that can be concluded is that there is some pathology present in the auditory system at or central to the inner ear. The presence of a sensorineural hearing loss does not tell us where along the auditory pathway the pathology is located; it only eliminates the outer and middle ears as possibilities. The pathology could be

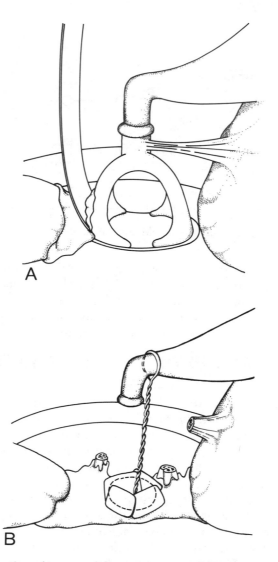

Figure 5.12.   Illustration of two surgical procedures on the stapes. **A**, Stapes mobilization; **B**, stapedectomy. (From Goodhill V (ed): *Ear Diseases, Deafness and Dizziness.* Hagerstown, MD, Harper & Row, 1979.)

affecting the sensory receptors within the cochlea, or the neural pathways leading from the cochlea to higher centers of the auditory system, or both the sensory and neural structures. In this context, then, "sensorineural" hearing loss is a very appropriate label.

The term *sensorineural hearing loss* is also an appropriate label for the hearing loss resulting from cochlear pathology for another reason. In cochlear pathology, the sensory receptors within the cochlea are destroyed. Exactly how this occurs depends on the specific etiology. Research conducted during the past 10–15 years suggests that the sensory destruction quickly becomes sensorineural damage. Once the hair cells within the organ of Corti are destroyed, a phenomenon known as retrograde degeneration occurs. Retrograde degeneration refers to the destruction of connecting anatomic structures located more central to the structure that was destroyed. Destruction of the sensory hair cells within the organ of Corti results in the eventual degeneration of the first-order afferent nerve fibers communicating with the damaged hair cells. Most patients with sensorineural hearing loss due to cochlear pathology, therefore, most likely have underlying damage to both the sensory (cochlea) and neural (nerve fibers) portions of the auditory system.

When a sensorineural hearing loss is observed, how do the audiologist and physician determine whether it is due to cochlear pathology or a problem lying further up the ascending neural pathways (called retrocochlear pathology)? As mentioned in Chapter 4, there are several steps involved in establishing the diagnosis. The case history taken by the audiologist or physician can provide some important clues as to where the problem might be located. The presence of other, frequently nonauditory, complaints, such as dizziness, loss of balance, and ringing in the ears (tinnitus), can aid the physician in establishing the diagnosis. A particular pattern of results from the basic audiology test battery may alert the physician to a probable underlying cause. The presence of a high-frequency sensorineural hearing loss in just one ear, for example, is a common audiometric configuration in some types of retrocochlear pathology. Finally, special tests can be performed on the patient at the physician's request. These tests may be auditory, in which case they are performed by the audiologist, or they may be nonauditory. An example of a nonauditory special test is electronystagmography (ENG), which tests the vestibular system and may also be performed by an audiologist. Another nonauditory test, one not performed by the audiologist, might involve some form of tomography. Tomography provides a visual image of the brain and brainstem structures. The most definitive auditory special test involves the measurement of the auditory brainstem response, or ABR. This test may also be administered by an audiologist. (The ABR was described in Chapter 3.)

Discussion of the special tests, auditory and nonauditory, that aid the physician in establishing the diagnosis is beyond the scope of this book. Suffice it to say that such tests exist and that the audiologist is frequently asked to perform them. Many types of cochlear and retrocochlear pathology, however, do produce a typical pattern of results on the basic audiologic test battery. The remainder of this chapter describes several of these pathologies and their audiologic profiles.

Cochlear Pathology

Prior to describing some specific etiologies that produce cochlear pathology, some general characteristics shared by most of the patients with cochlear pathology are noteworthy. First, for the most part, studies of human cadavers have revealed a close correspondence between the location of the damage along the length of the cochlea and the resulting audiometric configuration. For example, if postmortem anatomic studies of a patient's ear revealed damage in the basal high-frequency portion of the cochlea, then a recent audiogram obtained prior to death would most likely indicate the presence of a high-frequency sensorineural hearing loss. Although there are exceptions, it is generally the case in cochlear pathology that the audiometric configuration provides at least a gross indication of the regions of the cochlea that were damaged by the pathology (Vignette 5.3). A high-frequency sensorineural hearing loss reflects damage to the basal portion of the cochlea, a low-frequency sensorineural hearing loss suggests damage to the apical region of the cochlea, and a broad hearing loss extending from low to high frequencies reflects an underlying lesion along the entire length of the cochlea.

In sensorineural hearing loss due to cochlear pathology, there is a close correspondence between the frequencies that demonstrate hearing loss and the region along the length of the cochlea that is damaged. There is a less certain correspondence, however, between the degree of hearing loss at a particular frequency and the degree of damage at the corresponding location in the cochlea. One popular conception is that sensorineural hearing loss of mild or moderate degree is due to destruction of the outer hair cells, while more severe hearing loss reflects damage to both the outer and inner hair cells. At present, however, the evidence supporting this view has been primarily anecdotal in nature.

There are also several perceptual consequences of sensorineural hearing loss due to cochlear pathology. Except for those with profound impairments, the most common complaint made by the patient with cochlear pathology is that they can hear speech but can't understand it. This may be especially true when listening against a background of noise. The patient with cochlear pathology also frequently experiences a phenomenon known as loudness recruitment. This phenomenon was discussed earlier, in Chapter 3. The hearing loss makes low-intensity sounds inaudible. Moderate-intensity sounds that are comfortably loud to a normal-hearing person may be barely audible to the person with cochlear pathology. At high intensities, however, the loudness of the sound is the same for both a normal ear and one with cochlear pathology. Let us assume, for example, that a pure tone at 2000 Hz having a level of 110 dB SPL is uncomfortably loud for both a normal listener and a person with cochlear pathology. The person with cochlear pathology, however, has a hearing threshold at 2000 Hz of 60 dB SPL, while that for the normal listener is 10 dB SPL. Thus, for the normal listener, the intensity of the tone has to be increased 100 dB to increase the loudness of the tone from "just audible" (threshold) to "uncomfortable." For the person with cochlear pathology, however, an increase in intensity of only 50 dB was needed to cover the same range of loudness (from "just audible" to "uncomfortable"). Loudness increases more rapidly in the ear with cochlear pathology than in the normal ear. This is known as loudness recruitment.

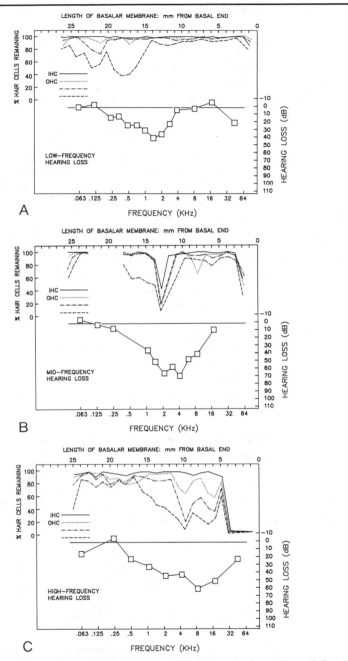

Vignette 5.3.   Illustration of the Relationship between Location of Cochlear Damage and Hearing Loss

The three figures accompanying this vignette illustrate the correspondence between the region of the cochlea that is damaged and the resultant hearing loss that is measured. The upper portion of each figure shows a "cochleogram" from three monkeys that were exposed to intense noise. A cochleogram depicts the percentage of hair cells within the organ of Corti that remain at various locations along the length of the cochlea after noise exposure. The percentages are determined after careful microscopic examination of the cochlea.

In panel **A**, the monkey was exposed to a low-frequency noise. This resulted in destruction of outer hair cells (OHCs) in the region roughly 15–25 mm from the base of the cochlea. Prior to sacrificing the animal to examine the type and extent of damage produced by the noise, the audiogram in the lower portion of the panel was obtained. A sensorineural hearing loss in the low and intermediate frequencies was produced.

When another monkey was exposed to a high-frequency noise (panel **B**), the cochleogram in the upper portion of the figure indicated that the damage appeared in the basal portion of the cochlea. Note that the audiogram obtained from the same monkey after the noise exposure and just prior to sacrifice (lower portion of panel **B**) revealed the presence of a high-frequency sensorineural hearing loss. As the damage to the sensory hair cells within the organ of Corti progressed from an apical (panel **A**) to a basal (panel **B**) region of the cochlea, the audiogram reflected the change as a shift from a low-frequency to a high-frequency sensorineural hearing loss.

Panel **C** shows a cochleogram and audiogram from a monkey exposed to a wideband noise. Note that the damage is much more extensive, affecting both the apical and basal portions of the cochlea. The damage, however, is most severe in the basal region. This is again reflected in the audiogram. The audiogram shows a broad hearing loss extending from low to high frequencies, more severe in the high frequencies.

(Adapted from Moody DB, Stebbins WC, Hawkins JE Jr, Johnsson L-G: Hearing loss and cochlear pathology in the monkey (macaca) following exposure to high levels of noise. *Arch Otorhinolaryngol* 220:47–72, 1978.)

The presence of loudness recruitment makes it very difficult to fit a hearing aid on a person with cochlear pathology. Low-level sounds need to be amplified to be made audible to the hearing-impaired person. High-intensity sounds, however, cannot be amplified by the same amount or the hearing aid will produce sounds that are uncomfortably loud to the wearer. Possible solutions to this dilemma when fitting the patient with a hearing aid are described in more detail in Chapter 7.

Finally, the patient with cochlear hearing loss may have accompanying speech abnormalities. Depending on the severity, configuration, and age of onset of the hearing loss, the speech may be misarticulated. In addition, if the cochlear pathology produces sensorineural hearing loss in the low and intermediate frequencies, the patient will typically use speech levels that are inappropriately loud, especially while talking without wearing a hearing aid. This is because the feedback that a speaker normally receives by bone conduction is not available to assist in regulating the voice level.

Now that we have reviewed some features shared by most individuals with cochlear pathology, the remainder of this section will examine several types of pathology. The pathologies described here are by no means an exhaustive compilation. In keeping with the general mission of this book, the pathologies described were selected because of their common occurrence either in the general population or among children.

High-Risk Factors

There are a number of complications that can arise prior to birth, during the birth process, or soon after birth that cause hearing loss. Many of these complications are factors included in the so-called high-risk register. The high-risk register is a checklist of conditions known to exhibit a higher-than-normal prevalence of hearing loss. These conditions include asphyxia, bacterial meningitis, craniofacial anomalies, hyperbilirubinemia, familial history of hearing loss, and low birthweight.

Viral and Bacterial Diseases

Severe viral and bacterial infections can result in varying degrees and patterns of sensorineural hearing loss. Infectious disease can be transmitted to the child by the mother in utero, a condition referred to as prenatal, congenital, or sometimes perinatal disease. These terms carry slightly different meanings yet are often used synonymously. The term *prenatal* refers to something that occurs to the fetus before birth. *Congenital* also implies before birth, but usually prior to the 28th week of gestation. Finally, the word *perinatal* pertains to a condition that occurs in the period shortly before or after birth (from 8 weeks prior to birth to 4 weeks after). A disease can also be acquired later in life, and this is usually referred to as a *postnatal* condition. The following discussion reviews some of the more common prenatal and postnatal infectious diseases known to cause hearing loss.

Prenatal Diseases

Many of the prenatal diseases are categorized as part of the TORCH complex, an acronym used to identify the major infections that may be contracted in utero. In the acronym TORCH, *T* stands for toxoplasmosis; *O* is for other; *R*, rubella; *C*, cytomegalovirus; and *H*, herpes simplex. Some have used the mnemonic (S)TORCH, where *S* stands for syphilis. Any disease of the (S)TORCH complex is considered a high-risk factor for hearing loss, and it is therefore important for the audiologist to have some general knowledge of these infectious conditions. Table 5.2 summarizes the (S)TORCH diseases and provides information about the expected hearing loss. In addition, audiometric patterns known to occur with most of the (S)TORCH agents are illustrated in Figure 5.13. Let us now briefly review these conditions.

Syphilis.   Syphilis is transmitted to the child by intrauterine infection from the mother. Syphilis may manifest itself anytime from the 1st to the 6th decade of life. When the age of onset is early (before 10 years), the hearing loss is a profound bilateral sensorineural hearing loss with sudden onset. With adult onset, the hearing loss is fluctuating and asymmetric and may appear either suddenly or gradually. Dizziness is also commonly associated with this condition. Figure 5.13**D** illustrates just one possible audiometric configuration associated with adult-onset syphilis.

Toxoplasmosis.   Toxoplasmosis is an organism that is transmitted to the child via the placenta. It is thought that the infection is contracted by eating uncooked meat or making contact with feces of cats. As noted from Table 5.2, about 17% of infected newborns exhibit sensorineural hearing loss. The hearing loss is typically moderate in degree and progressive (Fig. 5.13**B**).

Table 5.2.
Clinical Manifestations Associated with the (S)TORCH Complex

Disease	Primary Symptoms	Prevalence of Hearing Loss (%)	Type and Degree of Hearing Loss
Syphilis	Enlarged liver and spleen, snuffles, rash, hearing loss	35	Severe to profound bilateral SNHL; configuration and degree varies
Toxoplasmosis	Chorioretinitis, hydrocephalus, intracranial calcifications, hearing loss	17	Moderate to severe bilateral SNHL; may be progressive
Rubella	Heart and kidney defects, eye anomalies, mental retardation, hearing loss	20–30	Profound bilateral SNHL—"cookie-bite" audiogram is common; may be progressive
Cytomegalovirus	Mental retardation, visual defects, hearing loss	17	Mild to profound bilateral SNHL; may be progressive
Herpes simplex	Enlarged liver, rash, visual abnormalities, psychomotor retardation, encephalitis, hearing loss	10	Moderate to severe unilateral or bilateral SNHL

Rubella. Rubella is perhaps the most well-recognized disease of the (S)TORCH complex. Rubella, sometimes referred to as German measles, infects the mother via the respiratory route. The virus is carried by the bloodstream to the placenta and to the fetus. If the mother contracts the virus during the 1st month of pregnancy, there is a 50% chance the fetus will be infected; in the 2nd month, a 22% chance; and in subsequent months, about a 6–10% chance. Some of the more frequently encountered symptoms are shown in Table 5.2. One of the symptoms is a severe-to-profound bilateral sensorineural hearing loss (Fig. 5.13C). The child will display a trough- or bowl-shaped configuration or a corner-type audiogram. Children with maternal rubella have been known to exhibit both conductive and mixed-type hearing losses, although such instances are rare.

Cytomegalovirus (CMV). CMV is easily the most common viral disease known to cause hearing loss. About 33,000 infants are born each year with CMV. Ninety percent of the symptomatic children who survive (about 20% die) will exhibit complications. One of the common complications is sensorineural hearing loss. The hearing loss ranges from mild to profound and can be progressive. An example of a severe-to-profound hearing loss is illustrated in Figure 5.13A. The virus is passed from the mother to the fetus via the bloodstream.

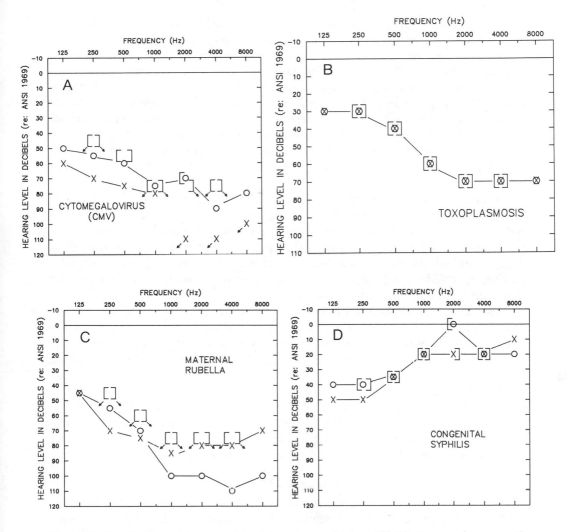

Figure 5.13.   Audiometric examples of **A**, cytomegalovirus (CMV); **B**, toxoplasmosis; **C**, rubella; **D**, syphilis.

Herpes Simplex Virus (HSV).   HSV is a sexually transmitted disease, and the acquired virus is passed on to the fetus in utero or during the birth process. Only 4% of infected infants survive without complication. Some of the complications of the disease include CNS involvement, psychomotor retardation, visual problems, and hearing loss. Sensorineural hearing loss occurs when HSV is contracted in utero.

Postnatal Infections

There are several postnatal infections that produce sensorineural hearing loss. The cochlear damage produced by these viral or bacterial infections appears to result from the infecting agent entering the inner ear through the blood supply and nerve fibers. Sample audiometric patterns for several postnatal conditions are shown in Figure 5.14. The following represents a brief review of those diseases that would be encountered most frequently by the audiologist.

Bacterial Meningitis.   Hearing loss is the most common consequence of acute meningitis (Fig. 5.14**B**). Although the pathways used by the organisms to reach the inner ear are not altogether clear, several routes have been suggested. These include the bloodstream, the auditory nerve, and the fluid supply of the inner ear and the middle ear. The prevalence of severe-to-profound sensorineural hearing loss among patients with this disorder is about 10%. Another 16% will exhibit transient conductive hearing loss. Interestingly, some patients with sensorineural hearing loss will exhibit partial recovery, although such a finding is rare.

Mumps.   Mumps is recognized as one of the more common causes of unilateral sensorineural hearing loss. The hearing loss is usually sudden and can vary in degree from a mild high-frequency impairment to profound loss. Figure 5.14**C** illustrates a case having a unilateral severe high-frequency hearing loss. Both children and adults are affected. Since it is not uncommon for this disease to be subclinical, children with hearing loss resulting from mumps are not usually identified until they first attend school.

Measles.   Measles is another cause of sensorineural hearing loss, affecting 6–10% of those infected with the disease. A typical audiometric configuration is a severe-to-profound bilateral high-frequency sensorineural impairment (Fig. 5.14**A**). It is also possible for patients with measles to exhibit a conductive hearing impairment.

Herpes Zoster Oticus.   The first symptom associated with this disease is a burning pain close to the ear. Shortly thereafter, eruption of vessicles (small sac-like bodies) occurs in the ear canal and sometimes on the face, neck, or trunk. Common symptoms include facial paralysis, hearing loss, and vertigo. The loss is usually a severe bilateral high-frequency hearing impairment.

Ménière's Disease

Ménière's disease is typically defined as a symptom complex affecting the membranous inner ear. It is characterized by progressive or fluctuating sensorineural hearing loss, episodic vertigo, and, frequently, tinnitus (ringing or buzzing in the ear) that varies in both degree and type. Some have added the symptoms of a feeling of fullness and pressure in the ear to the classic signs associated with this disorder. The most commonly reported etiologies of Ménière's disease include allergies, adrenal-pituitary insufficiency, vascular insufficiency, hypothyroidism, and even psychologic disorders.

Vertigo is considered the most characteristic symptom of Ménière's disease. It can occur in attacks that are extremely severe, lasting anywhere from a few minutes to several days. In its more severe forms, the vertigo can be accompanied by extreme nausea and vomiting.

Tinnitus, a ringing sound in the ears, often precedes an episode and subsequently serves as a warning signal for an impending attack. The tinnitus usually increases as the hearing loss associated with the disease increases. Most patients with Ménière's disease describe their tinnitus as a low-pitched narrow band of noise, much like a roaring sound.

The audiologic manifestation associated with this disease is most often char-

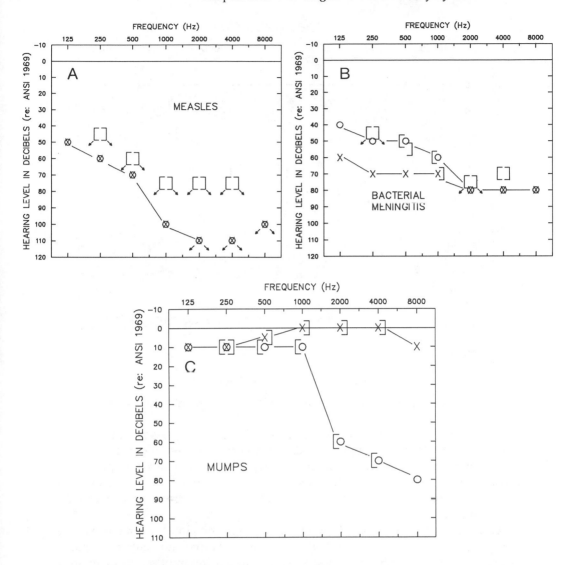

Figure 5.14. Audiometric examples of **A**, measles; **B**, bacterial meningitis; and **C**, mumps.

acterized by a low-frequency, sometimes fluctuating, sensorineural hearing impairment (Fig. 5.15). Although it has long been assumed that the disease is most often unilateral, estimates of bilateral involvement range from about 5 to 60%. In the later stages of the disease, the fluctuating nature of the hearing loss decreases, and the high frequencies become more involved. Typically, one sees good word-recognition scores and special auditory test results consistent with a cochlear lesion.

Ototoxic Drugs

A negative side effect of some antibiotic drugs is the production of severe high-frequency sensorineural hearing loss. A group of antibiotics known as

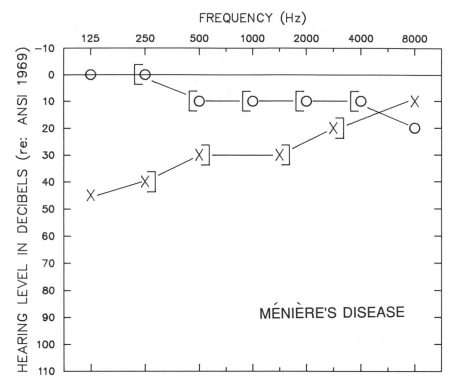

Figure 5.15. Audiometric examples of hearing loss due to Ménière's disease.

aminoglycosides are particularly hazardous. This group, also commonly referred to as the "mycin" drugs, includes streptomycin, neomycin, kanamycin, and gentamicin. A variety of factors can determine whether hearing loss is produced in a specific patient. These factors include the drug dosage, the susceptibility of the patient, and the simultaneous or previous use of other ototoxic agents.

Ototoxic antibiotics reach the inner ear through the bloodstream. The resulting damage is greater in the base of the cochlea, and outer hair cells are typically the primary targets, with only limited damage appearing in other cochlear structures. As shown in Figure 5.16, this results in an audiometric pattern of moderate-to-severe high-frequency sensorineural hearing loss in both ears.

Some ototoxic drugs cause a temporary or reversible hearing loss. Perhaps the most common such substance is aspirin. When taken in large amounts, aspirin can produce a mild-to-moderate temporary sensorineural hearing loss.

Noise-Induced Hearing Loss

Exposure to intense sounds can result in temporary or permanent hearing loss. Whether or not a hearing loss actually results from exposure to the intense sound again depends on several factors. These factors include the acoustic characteristics of the sound, such as its intensity, duration, and frequency content (amplitude spectrum), the length of the exposure, and the susceptibility of the individual.

When the intense sound is a broad-band noise, such as might be found in

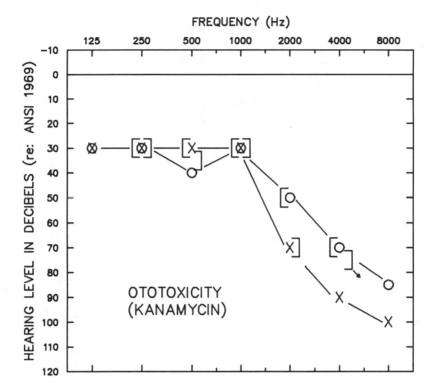

Figure 5.16.   Audiometric example of hearing loss due to ototoxicity.

industrial settings, a characteristic audiometric pattern emerges following the exposure. This audiometric configuration is shown in Figure 5.17. It is frequently referred to as a "4k notch," which reflects the sharp dip in the audiogram at 4 kHz. More detailed measurements of the hearing loss produced by exposure to broad-band noise reveal that the notch in the audiogram is as likely to appear at 3 or 6 kHz as at 4 kHz. Because 3 and 6 kHz are not routinely included in audiometric testing, however, the notch is less frequently observed at these two frequencies. This same "4k notch" configuration is observed both in temporary hearing loss following brief exposures to broad-band noise and in permanent hearing loss following prolonged exposure to such noise.

Many theories exist as to why the region around 4 kHz appears to be more susceptible to the damaging effects of broad-band noise. One theory is that, although the noise itself may be broad band, with roughly equal amplitude at all frequencies, the outer ear and ear canal resonances (see Chapter 3) have amplified the noise in the 2–4 kHz region by the time the noise reaches the inner ear. Thus, this region shows the greatest hearing loss. Other theories suggest that the region of the cochlea associated with 4 kHz is more vulnerable to damage due to differences in cochlear mechanics, cochlear metabolism, or cochlear blood supply. Whatever the underlying mechanism, damage is greatest in that region of the cochlea associated with 4 kHz. The damage again appears to be more marked in the outer hair cells, although this can vary with the acoustic characteristics of the noise.

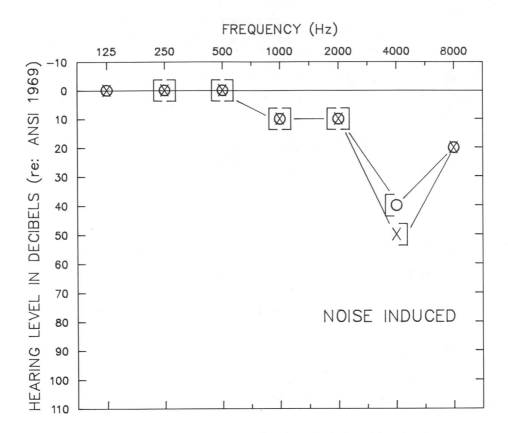

Figure 5.17.   Audiometric pattern associated with noise-induced hearing loss.

Presbycusis

Beyond about age 50 years, hearing sensitivity deteriorates progressively, especially in the high frequencies. The progression is somewhat more rapid for men than for women. Figure 5.18 shows the progression of hearing loss in both men and women as a function of age. The more rapid decline of hearing with age in men may not reflect differences in aging per se, but may reflect their more frequent participation in noisy recreational activities such as hunting, snowmobiling, or operating power tools (lawn mowers, chain saws, table saws, etc.).

The data in Figure 5.18 suggest that aging results in a sloping high-frequency sensorineural hearing loss that gets progressively more severe with advancing age. It should be noted, however, that audiometric configurations other than sloping ones can be observed in the aged. The sloping high-frequency audiogram described above is typical of the most common types of presbycusis, known as sensory and neural presbycusis. At least two other types of presbycusis have been described. These are referred to as metabolic and mechanical presbycusis and are generally associated with flat and very gradually sloping audiometric configurations, respectively. As mentioned, however, these configurations are much less common.

As shown in Figures 5.16, 5.17, and 5.18, the audiometric configurations

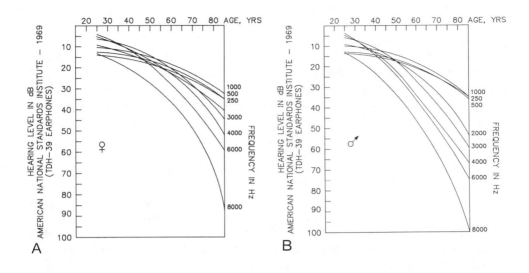

Figure 5.18. Illustration of hearing loss progression as a function of age in **A**, women; **B**, men. (Adapted from Lebo CP, Reddell RC: The presbycusis component in occupational hearing loss. *Laryngoscope* 82:1399–1409, 1972).

associated with ototoxic antibiotics, noise-induced hearing loss, and sensory or neural presbycusis are all very similar. In all three cases, a bilateral high-frequency sensorineural hearing loss is usually observed. The underlying cochlear damage is also very similar, with the basal high-frequency region of the cochlea being the main area of destruction and the outer hair cells being primarily affected. Accompanying retrograde destruction of first-order afferent nerve fibers is also typically observed, as is usually the case in cochlear pathology.

Degenerative changes associated with aging have also been observed in the brainstem and cortical areas of the ascending auditory pathway. These central changes can seriously compound the communicative impairment experienced by the elderly person with sensorineural hearing loss.

Retrocochlear Pathology

Retrocochlear pathology refers to damage to nerve fibers along the ascending auditory pathways from the internal auditory meatus to the cortex. Most often a tumor is involved, although not always, as in the case of multiple sclerosis (MS).

In many cases, the auditory manifestations of the retrocochlear pathology are subtle. Frequently, for example, no hearing loss is measured for pure tones. The possibility that a tumor along the auditory pathway will fail to produce measurable hearing loss for pure tones can be understood when one recalls the multiple paths by which information ascends through the brainstem within the auditory system (Chapter 3). Recall that after the first-order ascending neurons terminated in the cochlear nucleus, a variety of paths were available for the neurally transmitted information to ascend to the cortex. Thus, if the tumor is located central to the cochlear nucleus, the information required for the detection of a pure tone can easily bypass the affected pathway and progress to the cortex.

For the detection of a pure tone, many of the brainstem centers located along the ascending auditory pathways probably serve simple relay functions and perform little processing of the signal. For more complex signals, such as speech, however, some pre-processing probably takes place in the brainstem prior to complete processing by the cortex. Still, in many brainstem and cortical disorders, speech recognition appears normal in quiet.

This appears to be due to the multiple cues available in the speech signal that assist in its recognition. Some of the cues processed by a brainstem or a cortical center can be eliminated from the total information reaching the cortex by the presence of a tumor without producing a misperception of the speech signal. The patient is simply using several of the remaining cues that are not affected by the presence of the tumor. If, however, the speech signal is degraded by filtering, adding noise, temporal interruption, and so forth, the cues of the speech signal become less redundant. Every cue in the speech signal is now needed for its correct recognition. Individuals with retrocochlear pathology located in the brainstem or cortex typically perform poorly on speech-recognition tests involving the recognition of degraded speech signals.

Again, a detailed description of retrocochlear disorders and the tests developed for their detection is beyond the scope of this book. Many special speech-recognition tests making use of degraded speech have been developed for application with this population. In addition, as mentioned previously, the auditory brainstem response (ABR) and other auditory evoked potentials are also of tremendous assistance in aiding the physician in establishing a diagnosis of retrocochlear pathology.

Retrocochlear pathology that occurs at the first-order afferent nerve fibers, unlike that occurring at higher centers along the ascending auditory pathway, typically does result in abnormal performance on the basic audiologic test battery. These tumors, referred to as acoustic schwannomas, acoustic neurinomas, acoustic neurilemomas, or acoustic neuromas, typically produce a high-frequency sensorineural hearing loss that is either unilateral or asymmetrical between the two ears (Fig. 5.19). Most patients will also complain of tinnitus on the affected side, and slightly more than half of these patients complain of dizziness. Speech-recognition performance may range from normal to extremely poor at moderate intensities, but it typically becomes poorer as speech level is increased to high intensities. Acoustic reflexes are usually absent or present at elevated levels when the affected ear is stimulated. A special test, known as acoustic reflex decay, measures the amplitude of the middle ear muscle contraction over time during stimulation by intense pure tones. Patients with acoustic schwannoma who have a measurable reflex threshold typically show pronounced reflex decay, especially when stimulated with pure tones at or below 1000 Hz. If several of the above mentioned audiologic results are observed, the patient should be referred for additional testing. This will most likely involve measurement of the auditory brainstem response and other special auditory and nonauditory tests.

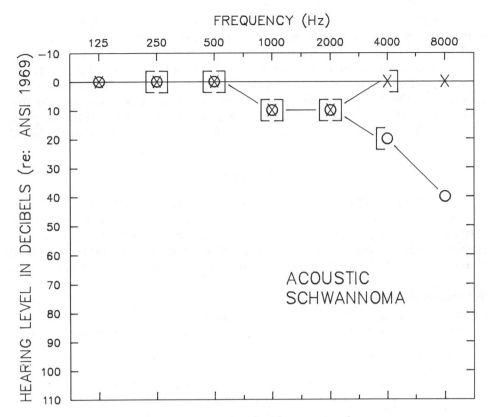

Figure 5.19.   Audiometric pattern associated with acoustic schwannoma.

NONORGANIC HEARING LOSS

The audiologist may obtain audiometric evidence of hearing loss when there is no organic basis to explain the impairment. Some of the terms commonly used to describe this phenomenon are nonorganic hearing loss, pseudohypoacusis, functional hearing loss, and psychogenic deafness. The cause for nonorganic hearing loss varies and is not clearly understood. Sometimes a patient may be purposefully feigning a hearing loss in order to gain a benefit (e.g., monetary compensation) or the patient may offer incorrect audiometric information because of a psychological disturbance. Whatever the reason, the audiologist must be able to determine whether a nonorganic hearing loss is present and, if so, what is the extent of the nonorganic impairment. Sometimes, a nonorganic hearing impairment will coexist with an organic hearing loss.

There are a number of audiometric signs that can alert the audiologist to the possibility of a nonorganic hearing loss. These signs include the source of the referral (e.g., insurance company referring because of a claim), an inappropriate behavior during the interview (e.g., exaggerated effort to speechread or to listen), and inconsistent audiologic test results (e.g., poor test-retest reliability). An obvious clue to nonorganic hearing loss is incompatibility between the pure-tone average and the speech recognition threshold (SRT). Recall from Chapter 4 that a relationship exists (± 10 dB) between the pure-tone average and the SRT. A person exaggerating a hearing impairment for pure tones cannot always provide equivalent hearing loss data for speech and thus will usually exhibit an SRT that is lower (softer) than the pure-tone average. Such a result should signal to the audiologist the possibility of a functional problem. There are numerous other special tests that have been developed for the purpose of detecting nonorganic hearing loss. However, detailed discussion of these tests is beyond the scope of this book. Those who are interested in learning more about these tests should refer to the Suggested Readings at the end of the chapter.

SUMMARY

The auditory system, marvelously complex and intricate, is nevertheless vulnerable to assault and damage from disease, trauma, genetic imperfection, extreme environmental conditions (i.e., noise), and aging. Many conditions affect both children and adults and can impact at all levels of the auditory system, resulting in conductive, sensorineural, or retrocochlear hearing problems.

References and Suggested Readings

Bess FH (ed): *Hearing Impairment in Children*. Parkton, MD, York Press, 1988.
Carhart R: Clinical application of bone conduction audiometry. *Arch Otolaryngol* 51:798–807, 1950.
Dahl AJ, McCollister FP: Audiological findings in children with neonatal herpes. *Ear Hear* 9:256–258, 1988.
English GM (ed): *Otolaryngology*. Hagerstown, MD, Harper & Row, 1976.
Fria TJ, Cantekin EI, Eichler JA: Hearing acuity of children with otitis media with effusion. *Arch Otolaryngol* 111:10–16, 1985.
Gerkin KP: The high risk register for deafness. ASHA 26:17–23, 1984.
Goodhill V (ed): *Ear Diseases, Deafness, and Dizziness*. Hagerstown, MD, Harper & Row, 1979.
Jerger J, Jerger S: *Auditory Disorders*. Boston, Little, Brown & Co, 1981.
Kavanaugh J (ed): *Otitis Media and Child Development*. Parkton, MD, York Press, 1986.
Lebo CP, Reddell RC: The presbycusis component in occupational hearing loss. *Laryngoscope* 82:1399–1409, 1972.
Moody DB, Stebbins WC, Hawkins JE Jr, Johnsson L-G: Hearing loss and cochlear pathology in the monkey (macaca) following exposure to high levels of noise. *Arch Otorhinolaryngol* 220:47–72, 1978.
Northern JL (ed): *Hearing Disorders*. Boston, Little, Brown & Co, 1984.
Shambaugh GE, Glasscock ME: *Surgery of the Ear*. Philadelphia, WG Saunders, 1980.
Shuknecht HF: *Pathology of the Ear*. Cambridge, Harvard University Press, 1974.

CHAPTER SIX

Screening Auditory Function

An important component of any comprehensive management strategy for the hearing impaired is an appropriate screening program. Screening is designed to separate those individuals who have an auditory disorder from those who do not in a simple, rapid, and cost-effective manner. Screening programs are intended to be preventive measures that focus on early identification and subsequent intervention. The objective is to minimize the consequences of hearing loss or middle ear disease as early as possible so that the disorder will not produce a handicapping condition.

The purpose of this chapter is to present information on screening for hearing loss and middle ear disease. The review will cover the general principles of screening, discuss screening procedures for hearing loss and otitis media used with different age groups, and recommend follow-up protocols for those identified as having an auditory disorder.

OBJECTIVES

Following completion of this chapter, the reader should be able to:

- Understand how screening programs can improve hearing care.
- Evaluate the efficiency of a screening tool and a screening procedure.
- Know the recommended screening procedures used to identify hearing loss or middle ear disease in different age groups.
- Understand the need for and the importance of follow-up programs.

UNDERSTANDING THE PRINCIPLES OF SCREENING

Factors That Determine Whether to Screen

How does one know whether to screen for the presence of a particular disorder? There are several criteria used in establishing the value of screening for a specific disorder. First, a disorder should be important. If left unidentified, the disorder should result in a significant damaging effect on an individual's functional status. It is also essential that the program be capable of reaching those who could benefit. Another important criterion is the prevalence of the disorder, or how frequently it occurs within a given population. There should be acceptable criteria for diagnosis. Specific symptoms of a disease must occur with sufficient regularity that it can be determined with assurance which persons have the disorder and which do not. Once detected, the disease should be treatable. Diagnostic and treatment resources must also be available so that adequate medical and educational follow-up can be implemented. Finally, the health system must be able to cope with the program, and the program must be cost-effective. It is generally accepted that hearing loss in people of all ages and middle ear disease in children satisfy these criteria and that screening for auditory disorders is justifiable.

What is an Acceptable Screening Test?

A screening test must be selected that will most effectively detect the conditions to be identified. A good screening tool should be acceptable, reliable, valid, and cost-effective. An acceptable test is simple, easy to administer, readily interpretable, and generally well received by the public. A reliable test should be consistent, providing results that do not differ significantly from one test to the next for the same individual. It does little good, for example, to have a screening test that the same healthy individual passes five times and fails five times when the test is administered 10 times in succession. Furthermore, the test should make it possible for examiners to be consistent in the evaluation of a response. Two different examiners testing the same person should obtain the same results.

Validity may best be defined by asking, "Are we measuring what we think we are measuring?" The emphasis in this question is on what is being measured. For example, a clinician who wants to identify middle ear disease has selected a screening test that involves the measurement of hearing. Such a test would not be valid because, while it might reliably measure a child's hearing loss, it cannot indicate the presence or absence of otitis media. Validity consists of two components: sensitivity and specificity. Sensitivity refers to the ability of a screening test to identify accurately an ear that is abnormal (whether from hearing loss or otitis media); specificity denotes the ability of a screening tool to identify normal ears. Thus, a valid test is one that identifies a normal condition as normal and an abnormal one as abnormal.

Finally, a good screening test is one that is cost-effective in relation to the expected benefits. Since the instruments designed to measure hearing loss and middle ear disease are reasonable in cost, the greatest expense is usually the salary for personnel. Other factors should be taken into consideration when estimating the expense of a screening program. These include the time required to administer the test, the cost of supplies, the number of individuals to be screened and rescreened, and the cost of training and supervising screeners. The following formula has been suggested to estimate the cost of a school screening program:

$$\text{Cost/child} = \frac{S}{R} + \frac{C + (M \times L)}{(N \times L)}$$

where C = cost of equipment in dollars; S = salary of the screening personnel in dollars per hour; L = lifetime of the equipment in years; M = annual maintenance cost in dollars; R = screening rate in children per hour; N = number screened per year. This formula could also be modified for determining the cost of an adult screening program.

Principles of Evaluating a Diagnostic Screening Test

In this section, we will cover some of the basic principles of how to assess the usefulness of a diagnostic screening test. Figure 6.1 sets the stage for understanding this diagnostic process. Our primary goal is to distinguish within the population at large those individuals who exhibit an auditory disorder ($A + C$) from those who do not ($B + D$). Within the group with an auditory disorder, subgroup A are those people with the disorder who test positive (true positives); subgroup C are those with the disorder who test negative (false negatives). Within the group without an auditory disorder, subgroup B are those persons without the disorder who test positive (false positives); subgroup D are all those persons without the disorder who test negative (true negatives).

Any diagnostic screening test must be evaluated against an independent standard, often referred to as a "gold standard." The results of the gold standard test are universally accepted as proof that the disease is either present or absent. In the case of hearing loss, pure-tone audiometry typically serves as the gold standard for any screening tool, whereas for middle ear disease the gold standard is usually pneumatic otoscopy or electroacoustic immittance. Figure 6.2 illustrates the way in which the characteristics of a diagnostic screening test can be evaluated against the gold standard. Toward this end, several terms and definitions need to be understood. First is sensitivity [$100A/(A + C)$]. (The factor 100 is introduced to convert the result to a percentage.) We have already learned that sensitivity refers to the proportion of individuals with the characteristic correctly identified by the test. If 100 subjects have a hearing loss and the test correctly identifies 75 of them, the sensitivity of the test would be 75%. Sensitivity is typically affected by the severity or duration of the characteristic. This is only logical in that, the milder an impairment is, the closer it is to a normal condition and the more difficult it is to distinguish from normal. However, the measure is not affected by prevalence. Another important measure is specificity, [$100D/(B + D)$], which refers to the proportion of individuals without the characteristic correctly identi-

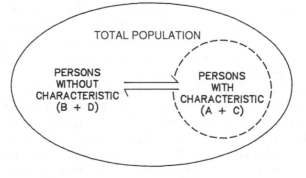

Figure 6.1.   Illustration of the diagnostic screening process. The purpose is to differentiate those who exhibit an auditory disorder in the population at large from those who do not.

Screening Test	Gold Standard Test: Characteristic — Present	Absent	Totals
Positive	A	B	A + B
Negative	C	D	C + D
Totals	A + C	B + D	A + B + C + D

Figure 6.2. A decision matrix illustrating the way in which to calculate operating characteristics of a screening test.

fied by the test. If, in a group of 100 normal subjects, the test identifies 70 as normal and 30 as abnormal, the specificity would be 70%. Like sensitivity, specificity is not affected by the prevalence of the disorder. The best screening tool will be one that provides the highest degree of both sensitivity and specificity.

It is possible to vary the accuracy of a screening test by altering the pass/fail criteria. A cutoff on a hearing screening test, for example might be 15 dB HL or 40 dB HL. A 15-dB HL cutoff will provide high sensitivity but lower specificity. This is because the 15-dB HL criterion will result in a larger portion of near-normal subjects being classified as hearing impaired. If a 40-dB HL cutoff is used, however, sensitivity will decrease but specificity will increase. The 40-dB HL cutoff will miss some of the mildly impaired near-normal subjects but will avoid misclassifying most of the subjects with normal hearing.

An important concept in any screening program is related to the prevalence of the disorder that is to be screened. Prevalence (derived from the word *prevail*) refers to the proportion of individuals in the population who demonstrate the characteristic [$100(A + C)/(A + B + C + D)$]. An important use of prevalence data is as a pre-test indicator of the probability of the disorder being present. For example, if the prevalence of hearing loss in the elderly is 30%, then when an older person walks into a hearing clinic you know that there is a 30% chance of hearing impairment before you conduct any tests. To illustrate how the prevalence of a disorder may be important to a screening program, consider the following two extremes. If 99% of the population has the disorder, it is easier to simply assume that everyone has it and treat it accordingly. In this case we would only be mistreating 1% of the population. If one in a million people have the disorder (prevalence = 0.0001%), then it may be safer and more efficient to assume that no one has it. Failure to screen for such a disorder would miss 0.0001% of the population.

In most hearing clinic settings, especially when screening for hearing loss, we need tests which yield maximum accuracy. The ideal test would be one that always gave positive results in anyone with a hearing loss and negative results in anyone without a hearing loss. Unfortunately, no such test exists. As a rule, one attempts to maximize the sensitivity and specificity of a screening test. This is done by evaluating different pass/fail criteria and test protocols in comparison to the gold standard. Examples of how to apply these general principles to actual screening data are shown in Vignettes 6.1 and 6.2.

Vignette 6.1.   Guidelines for Calculating the Operating Characteristics of a Screening Tool

Let us now go through the step-by-step procedures for calculating the characteristics of a screening tool. To assist in this process, some screening data are presented below. The gold standard was pure-tone audiometry. In this example, a total of 99 patients were screened and then tested using pure-tone audiometry. It is noted that 47 patients failed the screening test, 27 of whom actually had a hearing impairment and 20 of whom did not. On the other hand, 52 patients passed the screening. Of these, the gold standard showed that three had a hearing loss and 49 did not. The prevalence of hearing loss in the population screened $[100(A + C)/(A + B + C + D)]$ is 100(30/99), or 30%.

• First, the sensitivity, or the percentage of valid positive test results, is calculated from the data. The formula for computing sensitivity is $100A/(A + C)$. When applied to our data, this gives 100(27/30) = 90%. This is excellent.

• Next, compute specificity, or the percentage of valid negative test results, using the formula $100D/(B + D)$. This results in 100(49/69) = 71%.

In this example, we see that the screening test appears to be a valid tool for the identification of a hearing loss, offering acceptable sensitivity and specificity values. Now, on your own, calculate the operating characteristics of a screening tool for the Example in Vignette 6.2.

| | | Gold Standard Test | | |
| | | Hearing Impairment Characteristic | | |
Screening Test		Present	Absent	Total
	Fail	27	20	47
	Pass	3	49	52
	Total	30	69	99

STATUS OF IDENTIFICATION PROGRAMS IN THE UNITED STATES

Screening Programs for Children

Identification programs for hearing loss have been implemented in the United States for various age groups including the neonate, the infant, the preschooler, and the school-age child. Despite the urgency for early identification, however, the majority of screening programs occur at the school-age level. It has been estimated that less than 1% of the newborn population is being screened with the high-risk register, even though this tool has been recommended for universal use for several years. Moreover, only 14 states mandate some type of neonatal screening. This is most unfortunate, especially considering the relatively high prevalence of hearing loss and the critical importance of the first 2 years for the development of speech and language. In addition, a large number of pediatricians are not familiar with neonatal auditory screening, nor do they recognize its importance. It has been estimated, for example, that only

---

Vignette 6.2. Computing the Characteristics of a Screening Tool Using Hypothetical Screening Data

Now compute the characteristics of a screening tool for the example shown below. For this example, compute prevalence, sensitivity, and specificity.

Example:

		Gold Standard Test		
		Hearing Impairment Characteristic		
Screening Test		Present	Absent	Total
	Fail	160	20	180
	Pass	40	180	220
	Total	200	200	400

How did you do? You can find the answers in the back of the chapter.

3% of children from 6 months to 11 years of age receive a screening test at their primary health-care source. While it is true that more reliable responses can be obtained from infants and young children than from neonates, there is the problem of locating all of the older groups of youngsters for the hearing test. Once newborns leave the hospital, it is not until age 5 years, at the kindergarten level, that these children are available for testing at one common location. Those few screening programs that do exist are conducted in day-care centers, well-baby clinics, and Head-Start programs. These programs, however, attract only a specific segment of children, primarily those from lower socioeconomic levels. Even if a massive national effort were made to screen all preschoolers at these various centers, a large percentage of children would still be missed. Yet screening the preschool child has several distinct advantages over the screening of newborns:

1. Children become easier to test as age increases.
2. Children with a progressive hearing loss and those whose hearing loss was not detected at the newborn screening would stand a good chance of being identified.
3. Hearing-impaired children who have recently moved into the community would have a chance of being identified.

Under our present system, children whose hearing loss was not detected at the newborn identification program or who moved into a community at preschool age are not identified until screening occurs in kindergarten. There is a critical need for a national effort directed at infant and preschool hearing screening programs in every state.

Screening programs are most often conducted in the school system because it affords easy access to the children. However, the availability and comprehensiveness of school screening programs vary significantly from one state to the next.

The incorporation of immittance screening programs is not as universal. It is estimated that at least 24 states incorporate immittance (tympanometry) as part of their screening procedures. Some of the problems associated with immittance screening on a mass basis are discussed later in this chapter.

Screening Programs for Adults

There are virtually no formalized hearing screening programs in the United States for adult populations. Screenings do occur, however, in the Armed Forces, and most communities conduct health fairs where individuals can have their hearing tested. Adult hearing screening programs are also known to take place at community health centers, retirement communities, and nursing homes. Interestingly, evidence suggests that the primary-care physician typically does not screen for hearing even if the patient complains of a hearing loss. There is a critical need for audiologists to educate both consumers and health-care professionals about the importance of hearing health care, including early identification and intervention.

Audiologists and other health professionals have failed to sensitize both the lay public and the educational and medical communities to the effects of auditory impairment on total development. The importance of *early* detection of hearing impairment and the effectiveness of the screening methods available are two concepts that have not been presented well to the educational or medical community. Until we begin to educate these other professional groups, we cannot hope to improve our present identification programs.

IDENTIFICATION OF HEARING LOSS

Screening the Neonate

The advantages of detecting sensorineural hearing loss as early as possible in young children are important enough to encourage the implementation of newborn screening programs. It has now been demonstrated unequivocally that children who receive intervention from the age of 3 years or younger show significantly better speech and language outcomes later in life. Early identification and intervention (the word *intervene* means "to come in and modify") also results in substantial cost savings. For example, a deaf infant who receives educational and audiologic management during the first years of life has a better than 50% chance of becoming mainstreamed into a regular classroom.

The screening procedures advocated for the newborn nursery have been controversial. The most effective and appropriate techniques have not yet been agreed upon. The National Joint Committee on Infant Hearing (a committee comprised of representatives from the American Academy of Otolaryngology, the American Academy of Pediatrics, the American Speech-Language-Hearing Association, the Council on Education of the Deaf, and the Directors of Speech and Hearing Programs in State and Welfare Agencies) recommended screening only those infants who were considered at high risk for hearing loss. A listing of the Joint Committee's high-risk criteria is shown in Table 6.1. Unfortunately, studies have demonstrated that, while this approach can identify some infants

Table 6.1.
Listing of the High-Risk Register[a]

---

1. A family history of childhood hearing impairment
2. Congenital perinatal infection (e.g., cytomegalovirus, rubella, herpes, toxoplasmosis, syphilis)
3. Anatomic malformations involving the head or neck (e.g., dysmorphic appearance including syndromal and nonsyndromal abnormalities, overt or submucous cleft palate, morphologic abnormalities of the pinna)
4. Birthweight less than 1500 grams
5. Hyperbilirubinemia at level exceeding indications for exchange transfusion
6. Bacterial meningitis, especially due to *Haemophilus influenzae*
7. Severe asphyxia, a category which may include infants with Apgar scores of 0–3 who fail to institute spontaneous respiration by 10 minutes and those with hypotonia persisting to 2 hours of age

---

[a]Adapted from American Speech-Language-Hearing Association. Joint Committee on Infant Hearing Position Statement. ASHA 24:1017–1018, 1982.

with hearing loss, many hearing-impaired children do not manifest any of the risk factors listed in the high-risk register.

Behavioral Observation Audiometry

A number of behavioral techniques have been advocated in the high-risk nursery for screening for hearing loss. These techniques make use of a high-intensity wide-band stimulus or a band of noise centered around 3000 Hz. The stimuli are presented while the infant is at rest in a crib. The child's behavioral responses to these stimuli are then observed or recorded. A common behavioral technique of this type used in neonatal nurseries is the Crib-O-Gram. This test uses a motion-sensitive transducer placed under the crib to detect the infant's responses to the high-level noise presentations. Even subtle respiratory movement can be identified with this device. Behavioral techniques, however, exhibit a number of limitations. The approach generally will identify only those children with the more severe forms of hearing loss. In addition, because of the sound-field approach, it is possible that children with unilateral sensorineural hearing loss will not be detected. Finally, there has been concern expressed about the sensitivity and specificity of this approach because the response is as dependent on the infant's motor state as it is on sensory ability.

Auditory Brainstem Response (ABR)

Auditory brainstem response (ABR) has been suggested as a reliable indicator of hearing sensitivity in infancy. The advantages of ABR for newborn screening include: (*a*) the use of less intense, near-threshold stimuli, making it possible to detect milder forms of hearing impairment; (*b*) the ability to detect both unilateral and bilateral hearing losses; and (*c*) the use of a physiologic measurement that is entirely dependent on a sensory response. Limitations to the technique include the cost and sophisticated nature of the instrumentation, the use of an acoustic click that makes the ABR primarily sensitive to only high-frequency hearing loss, and the fact that the ABR is not a conscious response at the level of the cortex (presence of an ABR does not mean the individual can hear). Nevertheless, the measure is considered to provide a good estimate of hearing status when used carefully, especially when one considers the limitations of the alternative procedures. Failure of an ABR screening in the intensive-care nursery requires that the child be retested later under more favorable conditions.

There is now available a new automated response system known as ALGO-1. This device is a portable, automatic, battery-operated, microprocessor-based ABR test. Its primary function is to screen handicapping hearing loss in newborn infants. This simplified and cost-effective system employs a template-matching algorithm to determine pass/fail. The technique appears to have considerable promise for utilization in the high-risk nursery but is in need of further investigation before it can receive widespread acceptance.

Screening the Infant and Preschool-Age Child

Identification Tests and Procedures

Selection of screening techniques will be dependent on the age, maturity, and cooperation of the child. Generally speaking, a test of localization in the sound field will be required for those children between the ages of 4 months and 2 years. Conventional audiometric screening using earphones can usually be employed with children 3 years of age or older. Children between the ages of 2 and 3 years comprise the most difficult group for which to select an appropriate test. Some of these children can be conditioned for traditional screening techniques, whereas others will require the sound localization test.

Infant and Prenursery Child (4 Months to 3 Years)

The use of such acoustic stimuli as the human voice, rattles, a teaspoon and cup, and the rustling of tissue paper are often suggested for eliciting a localized (head turn) response. The child is placed on the parent's lap and various stimuli are presented about 2 feet from either ear. If the child fails to localize the signal, a rescreening is recommended. A second failure results in a third test 1 week later. If the child again fails the test, a complete diagnostic examination is conducted.

Sometimes delays in speech/language development are the most sensitive and valid indicators of hearing impairment among preschool children. It has been suggested that primary-care physicians and other allied health personnel screen young children for hearing loss simply by asking the parent three basic questions: (*a*) How many different words do you estimate your child uses? Is it 100 words, 500 words, or ?; (*b*) What is the length of a typical sentence that your child uses? Is it single words, two words, full sentences, or ?; and (*c*) How clear is your child's speech to a friend or neighbor? Would they understand 10%, 50%, 90%, or ? A general guide for referring children with a speech delay is offered in Vignette 6.3.

A more formalized test that probes for delays in speech/language development is known as the Early Language Milestone Scale (ELM). The ELM was designed primarily for physicians and other health-care professionals. It is considered to be a simple, rapid, cost-effective means of screening for communication disorders in children from 0 to 36 months of age; however, it is most sensitive at 24 months of age and higher. The test is a combination of parental report, direct testing, and incidental observation. Important for the primary-care physician is the fact that the test takes only 1–5 minutes to administer. Sensitivity values as high as 97% and specificity values as high as 93% have been reported when using

---

Vignette 6.3.   Referral Guidelines for Children with "Speech" Delay[a]

12 Months
No differentiated babbling or vocal imitation

18 Months
No use of single words

24 Months
Single-word vocabulary of ≤ 10 words

30 Months
Fewer than 100 words, no evidence of two-word combinations, unintelligible

36 Months
Fewer than 200 words, no use of telegraphic sentences, clarity < 50%

48 Months
Fewer than 600 words, no use of simple sentences, clarity < 80%

---

[a]From Matkin ND: Early recognition and referral of hearing-impaired children. *Pediatrics in Review* 6:151–156, 1984.

---

the ELM with preschool-age children. More representative values for sensitivity and specificity of the ELM are 65–70% and 65–75%, respectively. Nevertheless, the concept of asking parents specific questions relative to speech/language development appears to be a viable alternative for determining the presence of hearing loss among young children.

Preschooler (3–6 Years)

When the child reaches 3 years of age, the more traditional hearing test with earphones can be used for screening. By means of a portable pure-tone audiometer, signals may be presented at various frequencies at a fixed intensity level. The child merely indicates to the examiner, usually by raising a hand, if a tone was perceived. The American Speech-Language-Hearing Association has recommended that 1000, 2000, and 4000 Hz be used as test frequencies. If immittance testing is not part of the program, the frequency 500 Hz should also be tested (assuming that background noise levels in the test area are acceptable). The Association further recommends a screening level of 20 dB HL for all frequencies tested. A lack of response at any frequency in either ear constitutes a test failure. Failures should be rescreened, preferably within the same test session, but no later than 1 week after the original test. The practice of rescreening can significantly reduce the overall number of test failures. Children who also fail the rescreening should be referred for a complete audiologic evaluation.

Procedural Considerations Specific to Preschool-Age Children

In developing a screening program at the preschool level, special attention should be directed toward the groundwork and orientation process that occurs prior to the screening. The success of any screening program is dependent, to a large extent, on the cooperation that is received from the teachers, the children, and the parents. All three of these parties must receive some type of orientation to or familiarization with the screening process that is to take place.

First, a letter should go to the teacher outlining the need for and the purpose of the screening program. The letter should also review the teacher's responsibilities in preparing the children for the screening. Some suggested prescreening activities that the teacher can use in orienting the children to the listening task are outlined in Vignette 6.4. Such activities performed prior to the identification program can help avoid wasted time during the actual screening. It is also most

---

Vignette 6.4.   Recommended Prescreening Activities

I

Objective: To introduce children to wearing earphones in hearing testing.
Materials: Old set of earphones (if possible) or set of earmuffs
Procedure: Let each child examine and wear the earphones. Talk about the headband and the muff.
Variation: Allow the children to put the earphones on each other's ears.

II

Objective: To prepare children for the hearing test.
Materials: Blocks, shoe boxes.
Procedure: Put a shoe box on the table. Demonstrate holding a block up to your ear. Have one child stand behind you and clap his or her hands. Drop the block in the box when you hear the clap. Have each child take a turn standing in front of the box with the child's back toward you. Tell the children to "listen very carefully" and drop the blocks into the box when they hear the clap.
Variation: Let the children be the "hand clappers."
Note: If a child does not seem to understand, guide the child through the activity until he/she can hold the block to the ear and drop it in the box without your help.

III

Objective: To prepare the children for the hearing test.
Materials: Blocks, shoe boxes, bell.
Procedure: Put a shoe box on the table. Demonstrate holding a block up to your ear. Have one child stand behind you and ring a bell. Drop the block in the box when you hear the bell. Have each child take a turn standing in front of the box with his or her back toward you. Tell the children to "listen very carefully" and drop the blocks in the box when they hear the bell.
Variation: Repeat the activity and ring the bell softly. Have the children take turns being "bell ringers."
Note: Encourage the children to listen for the "soft" or "little" sound of the bell as preparation for the hearing test sounds that will be very soft.

helpful to provide the teacher with a list of the screening responsibilities of those individuals who will be conducting the screening, as well as of those who will be receiving the screening. This list will serve as an excellent guide and provide the teacher and/or administrator with a better understanding of the entire screening process from start to finish (Vignette 6.5). Finally, included in the packet of materials should be a sample letter to go to the parents of each child. The letter should explain the screening program so that the parents will understand the value of screening and be supportive of the screening process (Vignette 6.6).

The person who will be responsible for conducting the screening program should visit the facility and meet with the teacher(s) and administrator(s). Together they should review carefully the sequence of the screening program and discuss any concerns they might have. This is also an excellent opportunity to review with the program officials the sites available for the screening. Needless to say, a quiet room is essential. Other considerations in selecting a testing site have been identified by others. These are:

1. The site will need appropriate electrical outlets (only three-prong outlets should be used) and lighting.
2. The site should be located away from railroad tracks, playgrounds, heavy traffic, public toilets, or cafeterias.
3. The site should be relatively free of visual distractions.
4. Ideally, the site should have carpet and curtains to help reduce the room noise.
5. The site should have nearby bathroom facilities to accommodate the needs of the children and screeners.
6. The site should have chairs and tables appropriate for small children.

Some other suggestions and hints for screening preschool children include the following:

1. One person should be individually responsible for ensuring that the children move through the screening process smoothly and that all children receive the test.
2. Arrangements should be made for the children to have name tags showing their legal names and nicknames.
3. All forms should be accurately completed prior to the screening date. Each child should have his or her own individual preschool record form.
4. When screening children between the ages of 3 and 6 years, it is wise to alternate age groups during the screening day—for example, 3-year-olds followed by 5-year-olds. Three-year-olds are much harder to test and take more time. Another factor to keep in mind is that the little ones tire more easily than older children and need to be screened earlier in the day.
5. Screening activities should run from 8:30 or 9:00 AM until 3:00 or 3:30 PM each day. Schedule a full day, even if it means adjustments of schedules and bus runs and special notes of explanation for parents.
6. At all costs, avoid changing screening sites in the middle of the day. Each time you must dismantle a screening site in one center, move, and reassemble in another site, you lose approximately 1 hour plus travel time.

Vignette 6.5. Sequence of Screening Responsibilities

Agency Providing Screening	Program Receiving Screening
Appoint a person to coordinate all screening activities.	Appoint a program representative to coordinate all screening activities.
	Prepare a list of all program centers or children needing to be screened.
Procure the list of all program centers or children needing to be screened.	
Establish personnel needs based on number of children to be screened. Secure the necessary personnel to successfully implement the screening.	
Organize a training session in the use of screening materials, test forms, and test protocol for the screeners.	
Establish mutual screening schedules including dates and times, allowing ample time to do the necessary pre-screening activities.	Establish mutual screening schedules including dates and times, allowing ample time to do the necessary activities.
Provide assistance in screening site selection, if needed.	Choose screening sites.
Mail the screening materials and preschool record forms to the recipients. Materials should be in the teachers' hands 3 weeks prior to the screening date so ample time is allowed for forms to be completed, parent release forms to be mailed, and training in the classroom to be conducted.	
Inform screening teams about dates, times, sites, and personal responsibilities. All pertinent information should be in writing and given to screening teams approximately 2 weeks prior to the screening date.	Inform teachers about dates, times, sites, and personal responsibilities. All pertinent information should be in writing and given to teachers approximately 1 week prior to the screening date.
Conduct screening according to established schedule.	Assist in screening as needed.
Provide assistance in contacting resource agencies for follow-up or serve as the resource.	Contact resource agencies for necessary follow-up for the children failing the screen. Obtain comprehensive speech and language evaluations, therapeutic management, and in-service teacher training and assistance.

Vignette 6.5 (Continued)	
Agency Providing Screening	Program Receiving Screening
Type and mail a preschool screening summary report indicating the results of the screening by individual names grouped by classrooms. This report should be completed by the screeners within 2 weeks after the screening date.	
	Receive and review the preschool screening summary report with teachers and staff.
Provide ongoing monitoring of the follow-up activities on all children failing the screening.	Actively pursue follow-up management on all children failing the screening.

7. If the children are to be away from their own building during their regular lunch period, make arrangements for them to have lunch at the screening site if possible.
8. If the agency where the screening is taking place has a speech clinician on staff, ask to have that person available to assist in the screening effort.

Screening the School-Age Child

The practice of screening school-age children has been in existence for more than 50 years, and all states conduct some form of hearing screening in the schools. The Joint Committee on Health Problems in Education (consisting of members of the National Educational Association and the American Medical Association) has described some primary responsibilities to be met by a screening program: an awareness of the importance of early recognition of suspected hearing loss, especially in the primary grades; intelligent observation of pupils for signs indicative of hearing difficulty; organization and conduction of an audiometric screening survey; and a counseling and follow-up program to help children with hearing difficulties obtain diagnostic examinations, needed treatment, and such adaptations of their school program as their hearing condition dictates.

Who is Responsible for the Audiometric Screening Program?

Health and education departments are the primary agents responsible for coordinating audiometric screening programs. Ideally, the state department of education should coordinate the periodic screening of all school children as well as provide for the necessary educational, audiologic, and rehabilitative follow-up. The state department of health, on the other hand, should coordinate the activities of identification audiometry, threshold measurement, and medical follow-up for those students who fail the screening tests.

Personnel

The personnel designated to conduct the screening tests have been nurses, audiologists, speech-language pathologists, graduate students in speech and hearing—and even volunteers and secretaries. To assure quality programs, only professionals trained in audiology should be used to coordinate and supervise hearing screening programs. Volunteers and lay groups can best be used in a supportive manner, such as in the promotion of screening programs. Certified audiologists or speech-language pathologists should serve as the administrators of screening programs and utilize trained audiometrists or technicians to perform the screening. Public-health nurses may serve as organizers and supervisors, but can be of most value in the follow-up phase of the program. A nurse's responsibilities might include: (*a*) counseling parents and children about the child's needs for medical diagnosis and treatment; (*b*) using all available facilities to implement diagnosis and treatment; and (*c*) coordinating information about the child and family with specialists in the health and education field.

Who Should be Screened?

It is not economically feasible to mass screen all children in the schools. A target population must be identified. Most programs have concentrated their annual screening efforts on children of nursery school age through grade 3. In

---

Vignette 6.6   Sample letter to Send Parents Prior to the Screening Test

Special arrangements have been made for your child and the others in your child's class to be tested for hearing. This test is a wonderful opportunity and we want to be sure that every parent knows all about it.

Certain learning problems don't ordinarily show up until later school years, when they are harder to remedy. If these special needs can be found early in the school years, the problem can often be solved before it really gets started.

We are very fortunate to have trained, qualified people who will be testing our children during school hours one day in the near future. The testing is provided without any cost to you. Your child will enjoy the "games" that check the ability to listen. There is everything to gain . . . and nothing to lose.

Because of the large number of children to be tested, the procedure will have to be speedy. Therefore our children will be taking what is called a "screening test," which doesn't draw any conclusions—just finds the children who may need more careful testing.

The majority of the children will pass with flying colors (and have an enjoyable day doing it). If any problem areas are discovered, someone from the center (school) will get in touch with you to make arrangements to check out the problem completely.

None of us likes to think that our child could have anything that stands in the way of learning. By taking advantage of this screening test, we can make sure. The earlier a problem is found, the less a problem it becomes.

If you have any questions, please contact us.

_____

Teacher

fact, all of these grades are recommended for screening by the ASHA guidelines. Following grade 3, children may be screened at 3- to 4-year intervals. By concentrating the screening efforts on the first 3 or 4 years, it is possible to still provide careful observation of other special groups of school children. The following groups of children require more attention than that which routine screening provides:

1. Children with pre-existing hearing loss;
2. Children enrolled in special education programs;
3. Children with multiple handicaps;
4. Children with frequent colds, or ear infections;
5. Children with delayed language or defective speech;
6. Children returning to school after a serious illness;
7. Children who experience school failure or who exhibit a sudden change in academic performance;
8. Children referred by the classroom teacher; and
9. Children who are new to the school.

Equipment, Calibration, and the Test Environment

An important component of any identification program is the audiometric equipment used in the screening. The equipment needed for individual puretone screening should be simple, sturdy, and portable. Most screening audiometers are portable and weigh as little as 2 or 3 pounds. The performance characteristics of these instruments must remain stable over time. An audiometer that does not perform adequately could result in a higher-than-normal false-positive or false-negative rate. Care should be taken to ensure that all of the equipment used in screening satisfies the national performance standards. Unfortunately, this is not always done. Audiometers used in the schools often fail to meet calibration standards. School audiometers should receive weekly intensity checks with a sound level meter, as well as daily listening performance checks. A very thorough calibration of all aspects of the audiometer should be conducted each year. It is also suggested that spare audiometers be available in case a malfunction occurs during a screening identification program.

Older audiometers will be most subject to instability and malfunction and should receive careful surveillance. Clinical audiologists who use these instruments for threshold measurement (following a screen failure) should know that the masking stimuli generated by many of these portable audiometers are often insufficient to produce adequate masking.

Once again, screening must be conducted in a quiet environment in order to ensure accurate measurements. Although some modern schools have sound-treated rooms or mobile units with testing facilities, most do not. Screening programs must be conducted in a relatively quiet room designed for some other purpose. Some helpful guidelines for selecting an appropriate room for screening have been outlined in the section on preschool screening. The allowable octave-band ambient noise levels for each test frequency recommended by ASHA are shown in Table 6.2. These ambient noise levels are measured using a sound-level meter with an octave-band filter. (See Chapter 2.)

Table 6.2.
Approximate Allowable Octave-Band Ambient Noise Levels (dB SPL re: 20 μPa) for Threshold Measurements at 0 dB HL (ANSI-1969) and for Screening at the ASHA-Recommended Value of 20 dB HL

	Test Frequency (Hz)			
	500	1000	2000	4000
Octave-band levels:				
For testing with ears covered by earphone mounted in MX-41/AR cushion (ANSI 3.1-1977)	21.5	29.5	34.5	42.0
Plus ASHA screening level re: ANSI-1969	20.0	20.0	20.0	20.0
Resultant maximum ambient octave-band noise level allowable for ASHA screening	41.5	49.5	54.5	62.0

Identification Tests and Procedures

During the more than 50-year history of identification audiometry in the schools, tests have been developed for the purpose of screening the hearing of young school-age children. These tests may be classified as either group or individual screening tests. Most of the group tests were designed in earlier years to save time by testing large numbers of children at once. These techniques have never achieved wide acceptance. The majority of screening programs in this country have opted to use individual screening tests. Group screening, as it exists today, has only historical significance.

Individual Screening Tests

It is generally accepted that the individual pure-tone screening test is the most effective approach to screening hearing. In 1961, a comprehensive monograph was developed by the National Conference on Identification Audiometry (NCIA) outlining general guidelines for individual pure-tone screening. These guidelines recommended that screening be conducted at frequencies of 500, 1000, 2000, 4000, and 6000 Hz and that the screening occur in a sound-treated environment.

More recently, the American Speech-Language-Hearing Association developed its own set of guidelines for pure-tone screening in the schools. The ASHA procedures were developed in recognition that sound-treated environments were not readily available in the schools. The ASHA guidelines differ from the NCIA recommendations in that: (a) it is not recommended that screening occur in sound-treated rooms; (b) test frequencies of 500 and 6000 Hz are not included in the recommendations; and (c) rescreening of all failures is recommended.

Screening Adult Populations

With the increased awareness of hearing loss in the elderly population, we have witnessed an increased interest in the hearing screening of adult populations. Unfortunately, in primary-care medical practices where most older adults are seen regularly, we find that they are seldom screened and referred for audiologic evaluation. There seem to be several reasons for this. First, the elderly accept their hearing loss as part of getting older and believe that there is simply no recourse for improvement. Second, it is found that primary-care physicians often fail to recognize the presence of a hearing impairment. Even when hearing loss is suspected or is reported to the physician, more than half the patients are not referred for follow-up audiologic services. It appears that the primary-care physician looks upon hearing loss in the elderly in the same way that our society at large does. Deafness is viewed as a common by-product of aging, and little value is seen in providing rehabilitation to the individuals affected by it. Those physicians who do screen for hearing loss rely on such techniques as the case history, or whisper or watch-tick tests, approaches whose validity or reliability have not been tested. Recent studies have shown, however, that primary-care practitioners will, indeed, screen for hearing loss if provided with appropriately validated screening tools and if they are convinced that hearing loss is important to the life quality of their patient. Again, just as with preschoolers, the task confronting the audiologist is one of educating and informing the public and the health-care community.

Pure-Tone Screening

There is no accepted standard or guideline for the identification of hearing loss in the adult population. Some clinicians have suggested that a pure-tone screening level of 20 or 25 dB HL be used for frequencies of 1000 and 2000 Hz and that 40 dB HL be used for 4000 Hz. Others believe that a 20- or 25-dB HL level should also be used for 4000 Hz. Unfortunately, there are no data to support the validity of a 20- or 25-dB HL criterion at any frequencies for screening adults. We do not know the sensitivity, specificity, and test accuracy of pure-tone screening when using 20 or 25 dB HL as the cutoff point. Some have suggested that hearing screening in the aged should be done at the test frequencies 1000 and 2000 Hz, with a level of 40 dB HL serving as the pass/fail criterion. Failure for two test conditions (one frequency in each ear or both frequencies in one ear) constitutes a test failure. Data using this guideline are presented later in this section. Regardless of the test protocol, it is advisable to rescreen test failures. The recommendations related to environment, calibration, personnel, and procedural set-up that were discussed above regarding the screening of children can be followed with some modifications for screening the adult population.

Several new tools have been advocated for screening the older adult population. One of these is the Welch-Allyn Audioscope, a hand-held otoscope with a built-in audiometer that delivers a tone at 25 or 40 dB HL for 500, 1000, 2000, and 4000 Hz. An illustration of the Welch-Allyn Audioscope is shown in Figure 6.3. To use the audioscope, the clinician selects the largest ear speculum needed to achieve a seal within the ear canal. A tonal sequence is then initiated, with the subject indicating the tone was heard by raising a finger. The audioscope is found to perform very well against the gold standard of pure-tone audiometry when using the 40 dB HL signal at 1000 and 2000 Hz. The sensitivity of the audioscope has been reported to be 94% and its specificity is between 72 and 90% for identifying a hearing impairment. In addition, the test has been found to have excellent test-retest reliability.

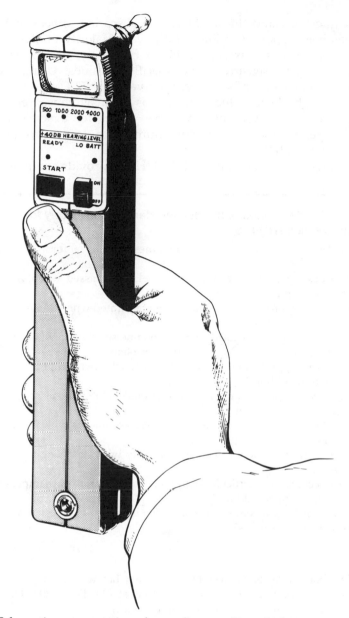

Figure 6.3.   Schematic representation of an audioscope (From Lichtenstein MJ, Bess FH, Logan SA: Validation of screening tools for identifying hearing impaired elderly in primary care. *JAMA* 259:2875–2878, 1988.)

Communication Scales

Communication scales represent another screening tool that can be used efficiently with the older adult population. A popular scale at present is the Hearing Handicap Inventory for the Elderly—Screening Version (HHIE-S). This screener is a self-report test that contains 10 items, five dealing with the social-situational aspects and five with the emotional aspects of hearing loss. A listing of the test questions and the instructions for scoring appear in Vignette 6.7. The test has been reported to identify the vast majority of elderly with high-frequency hearing losses exceeding 40 dB HL in the better ear. Again, this tool yields acceptable sensitivity and specificity values. Using a cutoff score of 8 (Vignette 6.7), one finds a sensitivity value of 72% and a test specificity of 78%. Although these values are not as high as those reported for the audioscope, they do represent acceptable values for a screening tool. The pencil-and-paper format and the low number of test items are additional advantages of the HHIE-S.

Even though the audioscope and the HHIE-S provide acceptable sensitivity

---

Vignette 6.7.   Illustration of the Hearing Handicap Inventory for the Elderly—Screening Version (HHIE-S)[a]

Enter: 4 for a "yes" answer; 2 for a "sometimes" answer; 0 for a "no" answer.

1. Does a hearing problem cause you to feel embarrassed when you meet new people?   _____
2. Does a hearing problem cause you to feel frustrated when talking to members of your family?   _____
3. Do you have difficulty hearing when someone speaks in a whisper?   _____
4. Do you feel handicapped by a hearing problem?   _____
5. Does a hearing problem cause you difficulty when visiting friends, relatives or neighbors?   _____
6. Does a hearing problem cause you to attend religious services less often than you would like?   _____
7. Does a hearing problem cause you to have arguments with family members?   _____
8. Does a hearing problem cause you difficulty when listening to TV or radio?   _____
9. Do you feel that any difficulty with your hearing limits or hampers your personal or social life?   _____
10. Does a hearing problem cause you difficulty when in a restaurant with relatives or friends?   _____

TOTAL   _____

HHIE-S scores may be interpreted as shown below. (Hearing impairment is defined as: (a) inability to hear a 40-dB HL tone at 1000 Hz or 2000 Hz in *each* ear; or (b) inability to hear both frequencies in one ear.)

HHIE-S Score	Probability of Hearing Impairment (%)
0–8	13
10–24	50
26–40	84

---

[a]Adapted from Ventry IM, Weinstein, BE: Identification of elderly people with hearing problems. *ASHA* 25:37–42, 1983 and Lichtenstein MN, Bess FH, Logan SA: Validation of screening tools for identifying hearing impaired elderly in primary care. *JAMA* 259:2875–2878, 1988.

and specificity values, the best test result is obtained when these two tools are used in combination. A summary of the screening characteristics of the audio-scope and the HHIE-S when used in combination is presented in Table 6.3. This table shows the sensitivity, and specificity, for each of the screeners alone and for the two instruments used in combination. Two specific pass/fail criteria seem to afford the most favorable outcome. These criteria include: (*a*) audioscope-fail and HHIE-S >8 or (*b*) audioscope-pass and HHIE-S >24. When these criteria are used, it is seen that the sensitivity is 75%, whereas the specificity is 86%. While there is some loss of sensitivity compared to that seen when either of the screeners is used alone, there is considerable improvement in specificity. This reduces the potential for overreferrals—an important factor when one is screening on a large-scale basis. Once again, as with most screening protocols, it is recommended that one use a retest before referral is made.

IDENTIFICATION OF MIDDLE EAR DISEASE IN CHILDREN
Electroacoustic Immittance

There is considerable interest in the use of electroacoustic immittance mea-sures as a means of identifying middle ear disease among children. Several factors have contributed to the interest in using immittance as a screening tool. Some factors relate to immittance in particular and others to screening for middle ear disease in general. These factors include the ease and rapidity with which immittance measurement can obtain accurate information, the relative ineffec-tiveness of pure-tone audiometry in detecting a middle ear disorder, the high prevalence of otitis media, and the growing awareness of the medical, psycho-logic, and educational consequences that may result from middle ear disease. Today this popular technique is used routinely, not only in audiology centers but also in public health facilities, pediatricians' and otologists' offices, and schools.

In 1977, a special task force studied the use of immittance measures in screening for middle ear disease. The task force recognized the potential value of immittance screening but concluded, after reviewing the available data, that mass screening with immittance was premature. The task force also recommended the screening of special groups of children, such as Native

Table 6.3.
Sensitivity and Specificity of Screening Tests in the Diagnosis of the Hearing-Impaired Elderly

	Sensitivity (%)	Specificity (%)
Audioscope	94	72
HHIE-S score		
> 8	72	77
> 24	41	92
Combined scores: audioscope fail *and* HHIE > 8, *or* audioscope pass *and* HHIE > 24	75	86

American, children, those with sensorineural hearing loss, developmentally delayed or mentally impaired children, and children with Down syndrome, cleft palate, or other craniofacial anomalies. The task force did not oppose immittance screening as such, but only universal (mass) screening on a routine basis.

In fact, recognizing that many screening programs were already in operation and that others were soon to be implemented, the task force developed procedural guidelines to be used in the screening of preschool- and school-age children. Some of the procedural considerations are outlined in Vignette 6.8.

A problem with immittance screening has been the difficulty of developing appropriate pass/fail criteria. The pass/fail criteria developed by ASHA and the special task force mentioned above have resulted in unacceptably high referral rates (32–36%). At present, the screening criteria known as the Hirtshals program appear to produce the best result. The program uses only tympanometry and does not include the acoustic reflex. At the first screen, all children with normal tympanograms are cleared. The remaining children receive a second screen in 4–6 weeks, and all cases with flat tympanograms are referred. Those children still remaining receive a third screen 4–6 weeks later. Children with normal tympanograms or tympanograms having peaks in the range of −100 to −199 daPa are cleared. Children with flat tympanograms or tympanograms with peaks ≤ −200 daPa at the third screen are referred. With the Hirtshal screening approach, sensitivity and specificity values are 80% and 95%, respectively. Moreover, the program yields an acceptable referral rate of only 9%. An

---

Vignette 6.8.   Some Recommended Procedures for Immittance Screening[a]

1. Tympanometry or a combination of tympanometry and acoustic reflex measurement can be used.
2. For eliciting the acoustic reflex, a signal of 105 dB HL should be used in the contralateral mode, or a signal of 105 dB SPL in the ipsilateral mode, or both.
3. Whether broad-band noise or pure tone is preferable as an eliciting stimulus for the acoustic reflex remains to be established. A pure tone between 1000 and 3000 Hz would be acceptable for this purpose. The stimulus should be specified.
4. Acoustic reflex measurements can be obtained either with the ear canal air pressure that results in minimum immittance or with ear canal air pressure equal to ambient pressure. The condition used should be specified.
5. For tympanometry, a 220-Hz probe tone is preferred. However, other low-frequency probe tones up to 300 Hz are acceptable.
6. For tympanometry, an air pressure range of −400 to +100 daPa is preferred. However, a range of −300 to +100 daPa is acceptable. Automatic recording should be used whenever possible, and the rate of air pressure change should be specified.

[a]Adapted from Harford ER, Bess FH, Bluestone CD, Klein JO (eds): *Impedance Screening for Middle Ear Disease in Children.* New York, Grune & Stratton, 1978, pp 5–7.

alternative approach to immittance screening is currently being developed by ASHA.

Acoustic Reflectometry

A relatively new and simple approach for detecting middle ear disease with effusion is known as acoustic reflectometry. This technique represents a non-invasive objective method and can reportedly be useful even if a child is crying or if there is partial obstruction of the ear canal.

The hand-held, otoscope-like instrument generates a 80-dB SPL probe tone that begins at a frequency of about 2000 Hz and increases linearly to about 4500 Hz in 100 milliseconds (0.001 s). The microphone in the device measures the combined amplitude of the probe tone and any sound waves reflected off the tympanic membrane (Fig. 6.4). According to the developers, the principle of operation is based on the consideration of one-quarter wavelength resonances. Briefly, an acoustic wave traveling in a tube will be completely reflected when it impinges upon the closed end of that tube. The reflective wave will completely cancel the original one at a distance one-quarter wavelength away from the closed end of the tube, resulting in zero sound amplitude at this point. Accordingly, the level of reflected sound is inversely proportional to the total sound. Greater reflection produces a reduced sound level at the microphone and suggests that middle-ear impedance is high—as in otitis media with effusion. The degree of reflectivity is numerically displayed on the otoscope. A reading of 0–2 denotes a clear ear, and a reading of greater than 5 implies higher impedance, as with effusion.

Studies on the acoustic reflectometer have reported mixed results; about one-half of the studies report excellent sensitivity and specificity values, and one-half report unacceptable values. Research, however, has been limited with this device. More research is needed before this screening instrument can receive widespread acceptance.

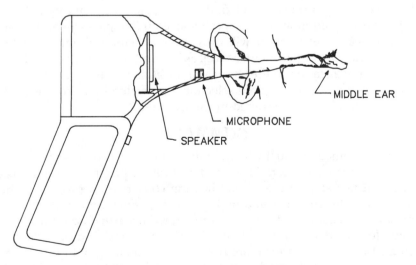

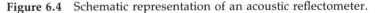

Figure 6.4 Schematic representation of an acoustic reflectometer.

FOLLOW-UP

Follow-Up Programs for Children

Screening is of little value if follow-up is not provided for the appropriate management of children who fail the rescreening. This aspect of the conservation program takes as much planning and effort as any other phase of the screening program. Under most circumstances, the screening coordinator will be the person responsible for the follow-up.

A child who fails the rescreen should receive a threshold test at the screening site as soon as possible. Within a few days following the screening, those steps essential to appropriate follow-up should begin. Letters should be sent to parents indicating whether their child passed or failed the screening test. For those children who failed the screening, the letter should also recommend that the child be referred for medical evaluation. About 6 weeks after the screening, an inquiry should be directed to the parents to determine whether the recommendations were followed.

Frequently the public-health nurse handles the responsibility of this phase of the follow-up program. In some states, audiologists and educators coordinate this activity. Following the medical examination, the child is referred to an audiologic facility where comprehensive testing and counseling occur. Parent counseling is an important aspect of the follow-up process and too often is overlooked by the supervisors of screening programs. Parents must receive special assistance and guidance in order to understand and cope with the prospect of having a hearing-impaired child. They must receive help before they can help their child.

Finally, the child will need to be referred to educational services that will be used for planning and placement. The follow-up is a lengthy and ongoing process requiring close coordination among all persons involved.

Follow-Up Programs for Adult Populations

If the screening protocol is failed, it is advisable for the individual to receive an otologic examination and a comprehensive audiologic evaluation. Needless to say, the hearing evaluation will provide information about the extent and nature of the hearing impairment, as well as determine whether the patient could benefit from amplification. If the use of amplification is warranted, the individual should be referred for hearing aid selection and evaluation. Procedures for this particular protocol will be outlined in the Chapter 7.

SUMMARY

We have defined and justified screening and discussed important considerations and techniques concerned with identification programs. Identification is an important first step in the overall hearing conservation program. The early identification of hearing loss and middle ear disease is the key to effective and appropriate management. There still is much to be learned about our screening programs for the identification of both hearing loss and middle ear disease. In particular, there is a need for more research on screening with immittance and acoustic reflectometry for middle ear disease in children. There is still only limited information available about the application of the latter technique as a screening device, and the audiologist, therefore, will need to keep abreast of new developments. Finally, it will also be important to determine the sensitivity, specificity, and test accuracy of pure-tone audiometry for the adult population when using a 20- or 25-dB HL cutoff point.

References and Suggested Readings

American National Standards Institute: *American National Standards Specifications for Audiometers*. ANSI S3.6-1969. New York, American National Standards Institute, 1970.

American Speech-Language-Hearing Association: Guidelines for acoustic immittance screening of middle ear function. *ASHA* 20:550–555, 1978.

American Speech-Language-Hearing Association: Guidelines for identification audiometry. *ASHA* 27:49–53, 1985.

American Speech-Language-Hearing Association: Guidelines for screening for hearing impairment and middle ear disorders (Draft: for peer review). *ASHA* 31:71–76, 1989.

Avery C, Gates G, Prihoda T: Efficacy of acoustic reflectometry in detecting middle ear effusion. *Ann Otol Rhinol Laryngol* 95:472–476, 1986.

Cooper J, Gates G, Owen J, Dickson H: An abbreviated impedance bridge technique for school screening. *J Speech Hear Disord* 40:260–269, 1974.

Coplan J, Gleason JR, Ryan R, Burke MG, Williams ML: Validation of an early language milestone scale in a high risk population. *Pediatrics* 70:677-683, 1982.

Coscarelli JE: *Selection of Testing Site*. Bureau of Education for the Handicapped Outreach Project. Grant no. G00701865, Project no. 444BH 70083. Nashville, TN, Urban Observatory, 1977.

Darley FL (ed): Identification audiometry. *J Speech Hear Disord* (Monogr. Suppl. 9), 1961.

Downs M: Early identification of hearing loss: where are we? where do we go from here? In Mencher GT (ed): *Early Identification of Hearing Loss*. Basel, S Karger, 1976.

Eagles EL, Wishik SM, Doerfler LG: Hearing sensitivity and ear disease in children: a prospective study. *Laryngoscope* (Suppl), 1967.

Harford ER, Bess FH, Bluestone CD, Klein JO (eds): *Impedance Screening for Middle Ear Disease in Children*. New York, Grune & Stratton, 1978.

Holmes AE, Muir-Jones KC, Kemker FJ: Acoustic reflectometry versus tympanometry in pediatric middle ear screenings. *Language, Speech and Hearing Services in the Schools* 20:41–49, 1989.

Kileny PR: ALGO-1 automated infant hearing screener: preliminary results. In Gerkin KP, Amochaev A (eds): *Hearing in Infants: Proceedings from the National Symposium*. Seminars in Hearing. New York, Thieme-Stratton, 1987.

Levitt H, McGarr N: Speech and language development in hearing-impaired children. In Bess FH (ed): *Hearing Impairment in Children*. Parkton, MD, York Press, 1988.

Lichtenstein MJ, Bess FH, Logan SA: Validation of screening tools for identifying hearing impaired elderly in primary care. *JAMA* 259:2875-2878, 1988.

Lous J: Screening for secretory otitis media: evaluation of some impedance programs for long-lasting secretory otitis media in 7-year-old children. *Int J Pediatr Otorhinolaryngol* 13:85–97, 1987.

Matkin ND: Early recognition and referral of hearing-impaired children. *Pediatrics in Review*, 6:151–156, 1984.

Melnick W, Eagles EL, Levine HS: Evaluation of a recommended program of identification audiometry with school-age children. *J Speech Hear Disord* 29:3-13, 1964.

Northern JL, Downs MP: *Hearing in Children*, ed 3. Baltimore, Williams & Wilkins, 1984.

Sackett DL, Haynes RB, Tugwell P: *Clinical Epidemiology: A Basic Science for Clinical Medicine*. Boston, Little, Brown & Co, 1985.

Schwartz DM, Schwartz RH, Daly UJ: Efficacy of acoustic reflectometry in detecting middle ear fluid. Presented at Audiology Update: Pediatric Audiology, Newport, RI, 1984.

Ventry IM, Weinstein BE: Identification of elderly people with hearing problems. *ASHA* 25:37–42, 1983.

Walton WK, Williams PS: Stability of routinely serviced portable audiometers. *Language, Speech, Hearing Services in the Schools* 3:36–43, 1972.

Weber BA: Screening of high-risk infants using auditory brainstem response audiometry. In Bess FH (ed): *Hearing Impairment in Children*. Parkton, MD, York Press, 1988.
Wilson WR, Walton WK: Public school audiometry. In Martin FN (ed): *Pediatric Audiology*. Englewood Cliffs, NJ, Prentice-Hall, 1978.

Answers to Problem in Vignette 6.2

Prevalence—50%
Sensitivity—80%
Specificity—90%

CHAPTER SEVEN

Amplification and Rehabilitation for the Hearing Impaired

Probably the most significant problem experienced by the hearing-impaired adult is difficulty understanding speech, especially against a background of noise. Individuals with severe or profound sensorineural hearing loss also have trouble hearing their own speech. This typically results in speech production problems as well, making the overall communication process even more difficult. The intent of rehabilitation for the hearing-impaired adult is to restore as much speech-comprehension and speech-production ability as possible. For the congenitally hearing-impaired child, however, the problem is more complicated since the symbols of our language system have not yet been learned. In these circumstances, the emphasis is on helping the child to acquire this complex language system and to use language appropriately so that communication skills might be achieved. The focus is more on habilitation than rehabilitation. That is, the objective is not to restore a skill that once existed, but to help the child develop a new skill, the ability to communicate. In this chapter, we will review different approaches for developing and/or improving the communicative abilities of hearing-impaired children and adults. This process is usually referred to as aural rehabilitation or aural habilitation. A central core of any rehabilitation/habilitation program is the use of a hearing aid, an amplification device designed to help compensate for the hearing deficit. A substantial portion of this chapter focuses on various aspects of amplification systems.

OBJECTIVES

Following completion of this chapter, the reader should be able to:

- List and describe the devices currently available to assist in the rehabilitation of the hearing impaired, including conventional hearing aids, assistive listening devices, classroom amplification, cochlear implants, and vibrotactile systems.

- Understand the basic components, function, and electroacoustic characteristics of hearing aids.
- Describe the general approaches used to select and evaluate conventional hearing aids.
- Understand some of the principles and techniques used in the management of hearing-impaired children and adults.

AURAL REHABILITATION/HABILITATION PROCESS

The aural rehabilitation process involves at least two phases. The first phase is the identification of the problem. Before an intervention strategy can be developed, one must know about the type and degree of hearing loss as well as the impact of the impairment on communicative, educational, social, or cognitive function. For the hearing-impaired adult, the measurement of the patient's audiogram, the administration of speech-recognition tests, and the use of self-report surveys or questionnaires can provide much of this information. Pure-tone and speech audiometry have been discussed previously (Chapter 4). Self-report surveys are often used to assess in detail the social, psychological, and communicative difficulties experienced by the hearing impaired. The Hearing Handicap Inventory for the Elderly—Screening version (HHIE-S), discussed in the previous chapter, is an example of such a survey, but in an abbreviated format. For the hearing-impaired child, additional assessment considerations might include the extent of parental support and the evaluation of skills in language, speech, auditory training, and speechreading (lipreading).

After the problem has been identified, the next phase of the rehabilitation process is intervention. For the hearing impaired, the nature of the intervention package is determined, in large part, by the results observed during the identification phase. Consider, for example, just the degree and type of hearing loss, ignoring other factors such as age and social/emotional difficulties. First, regarding type of hearing loss, the most appropriate candidates for amplification are those with sensorineural hearing loss. Occasionally, individuals with chronic conductive hearing loss not amenable to medical or surgical intervention will be fitted with a hearing aid. Most often, though, the individual with sensorineural hearing loss due to cochlear pathology is the type of patient fitted with a rehabilitative device, such as a hearing aid.

Generally, as the degree of sensorineural hearing loss increases, speech-understanding difficulties increase. The need for intervention increases in proportion to the degree of speech-understanding difficulty. Thus, those with mild hearing loss (pure-tone average of 20–30 dB HL) generally have less need for intervention than those with profound hearing loss (>85 dB HL). Conventional hearing aids provide the greatest benefit to those hearing-impaired persons having average hearing loss between 40 and 85 dB HL. For milder amounts of hearing loss, the difficulties experienced and the need for intervention are not great enough for full-time use of a conventional hearing aid. Part-time use of a hearing aid, or another type of device known as an assistive listening device, is usually recommended for these patients. For the profoundly impaired, on the other hand, the difficulties in communicating and the need for intervention are great. Unfortunately, the conventional hearing aid is of limited benefit in such cases. For those patients with profound impairments, alternative devices, such as vibrotactile systems and cochlear implants, are sometimes explored. Currently, however, high-powered conventional aids are still the most common alternative for the profoundly impaired. Because of the limited benefit amplification provides for this group, though, the fitting of the hearing aid is usually accompanied by extensive training in several areas, including speechreading (lipreading), auditory training, and/or manual communication (finger spelling and sign language).

Consider also the time of onset of the hearing loss. Of course, the intervention approach will be much different for a congenitally hearing-impaired child than for someone who acquired the hearing loss later in life (after communication has developed). With a congenital onset, the emphasis will focus on such critical issues as early amplification, parental guidance, and a comprehensive habilitation package designed to facilitate communication development.

In summary, the intervention phase of aural rehabilitation/habilitation typically begins with the selection and fitting of an appropriate rehabilitative device, such as a hearing aid. This is followed by extensive training in communicative skills with the device.

Many of the procedures used in the identification phase of the rehabilitation process have been reviewed in earlier chapters. In this chapter, the focus is placed on the intervention phase. The remainder of this chapter is divided into three sections. The first section reviews many of the rehabilitative devices available, with emphasis placed on the conventional hearing aid. Methods of selecting and evaluating hearing aids are also reviewed in the first section. The final two sections review training methods and philosophies for rehabilitation/ habilitation of children and adults.

AMPLIFICATION FOR THE HEARING IMPAIRED

Classification of Conventional Amplification

There are five basic types of hearing aid available today. These are: (1) body aid; (2) eyeglass aid; (3) behind-the-ear (BTE) aid; (4) in-the-ear (ITE) aid; and (5) in-the-canal (ITC) aid. Figure 7.1 shows each type of instrument. When electroacoustic hearing aids were first developed several decades ago, the body aid was the only type available. In the ensuing years, the other types of instruments were developed, with BTE hearing aids being the most common in the 1970s. During the 1980s, the trend has been for ITEs to capture an increasingly larger portion of the hearing aid market. This trend over the past decade is summarized in Figure 7.2. The increasing popularity of the ITE and ITC hearing aids is a result of both consumer pressures to improve the cosmetic appeal of the devices and rapid developments in the field of electronics. High-fidelity electronic components and the batteries to power them have been drastically reduced in size, making the in-the-ear devices possible.

Operation Of Amplification Systems

Components and Function

Although the outer physical characteristics of the types of hearing aids shown in Figure 7.1 differ, the internal features are very similar. The hearing aid, for example, is referred to as an electroacoustic device. It converts the acoustic signal, such as a speech sound, into an electrical signal. The device then

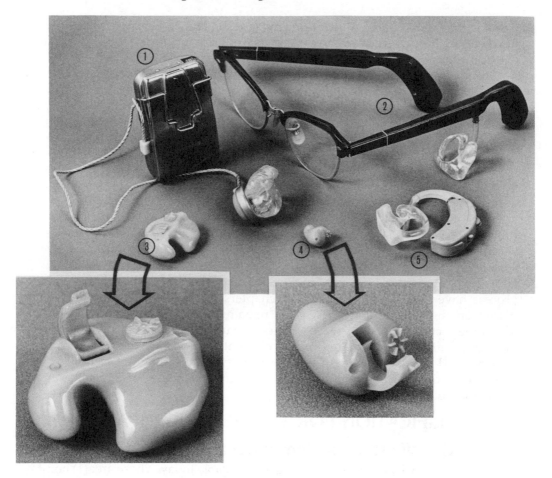

Figure 7.1.   Illustration of the different types of hearing aids. 1, body aid; 2, eyeglass; 3, in-the-ear aid; 4, in-the-canal aid; and 5, behind-the-ear aid.

manipulates the electrical signal in some way, converts the electrical signal back to an acoustic one, and then delivers it to the ear canal of the wearer. A microphone is used to convert the acoustic signal into an electrical signal. The electrical signal is usually amplified or made larger within the hearing aid. It may also be filtered to eliminate high or low frequencies from the signal. A tiny loudspeaker, usually referred to as a receiver, converts the amplified electrical signal back into a sound wave. Up to this point, the hearing aid could be thought of as a miniature public-address system with a microphone, amplifier, and loudspeaker. Unlike a public-address system, though, the hearing aid is designed to help a single person, the hearing aid wearer, receive the amplified speech. The microphone is positioned somewhere on the hearing-aid wearer, and the amplified sound from the receiver is routed directly to the wearer's ear. For in-the-ear and in-the-canal hearing aids, the sound wave is routed from the receiver to the ear canal by a small piece of tubing within the instrument. For the other types of hearing aids, an earmold is needed. The earmold is made of a synthetic plastic or rubber-like material from an impression made of the outer ear and ear canal. The earmold

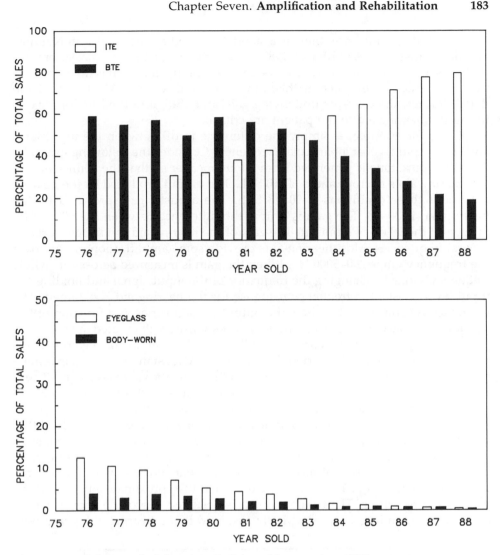

Figure 7.2. Sales trends for various hearing aid types since 1975.

is custom-made for the patient's ear and allows the output of the hearing aid to be coupled to the patient's ear canal. As a result, only the patient receives the louder sound and not a group of people, as with a public-address system.

Electroacoustic Characteristics of Hearing Aids

The primary purpose of the hearing aid is to make speech that is inaudible to the hearing-impaired person audible, and to do so without causing discomfort. Modern-day conventional hearing aids have several electroacoustic characteristics that are used to describe the hearing aid's performance. Probably the two most important of these characteristics are the amount of amplification provided, referred to as the gain of the instrument, and the maximum possible sound pressure level that can be produced, referred to as the saturation sound pressure level (SSPL). Currently, there are several ways in which these characteristics can be measured. For instance, there is a standard issued by the American National Standards Institute, ANSI S3.22–1987, which describes a set of measurements that must be made on all hearing aids sold in the United States. It is not necessary in an introductory text such as this, however, to review the ANSI standard in detail. Rather, the concepts underlying gain and SSPL and their importance in fitting the hearing aid to the patient are critical.

Gain, for example, is simply the difference in dB between the input level and the output level at a particular frequency. Consider the following example. A 500-Hz pure tone is generated from a loudspeaker so that the sound level at the hearing aid's microphone is 60 dB SPL. The output produced by the hearing aid under these conditions is 90 dB SPL. The acoustic gain provided by the hearing aid is 30 dB. The gain is simply the difference between the 60-dB SPL input and the 90-dB SPL output. The gain of the hearing aid can be measured at several frequencies. Most hearing aids provide some amplification or gain over the frequency range 200–5000 Hz. When the gain is measured across this whole frequency range by changing the frequency of the input signal and holding the input level constant, a frequency response for the hearing aid is obtained. The frequency response displays how the output or gain varies as a function of frequency. The concepts of gain and frequency response are illustrated in Figure 7.3. Because the gain is seldom constant at all frequencies, an average gain value is frequently calculated and reported. In the current ANSI standard, the gain is measured at three frequencies, 1000, 1600, and 2500 Hz, and the values averaged. These frequencies are used because of their importance to speech understanding and because the hearing aid usually has its greatest output in this frequency region.

A feature shared by all types of hearing aids is a volume control wheel that allows the user to adjust the gain of the hearing aid. The frequency response of the hearing aid can be measured with the position of the volume control varied. Usually, at least two sets of measurements are obtained: one with the volume control in the full-on position, and one designed to approximate a typical or "as worn" volume setting. The volume control is designed to provide approximately a 30-dB variation in gain. It is typically assumed that a hearing aid wearer will

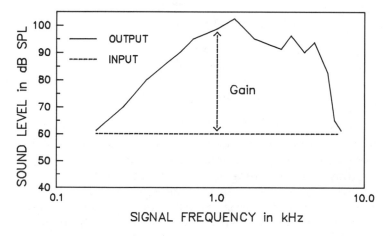

Figure 7.3.   Illustration of the calculation of hearing aid gain. The *output* curve represents the frequency response of the hearing aid for a constant 60-dB *input*.

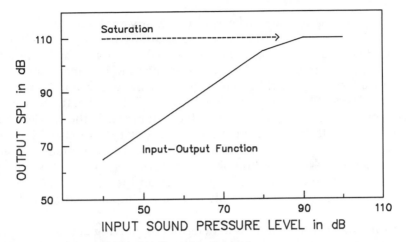

Figure 7.4. Input-output function for a hearing aid.

select a volume setting about in the middle of this 30-dB range—that is, about 15 dB below the full-on position. If the frequency response is measured with the volume control of the hearing aid in the full-on position, the gain is referred to as "full-on" gain. When the volume control is in the middle of the usable range, the gain approximates "use" gain, or "as worn" gain.

As mentioned, a second fundamental electroacoustic characteristic of the hearing aid is the saturation sound pressure level (SSPL). The measurement of SSPL is designed to determine the maximum possible acoustic output of the hearing aid. Consequently, a high level input signal is used (90 dB SPL), and the volume control is set to the full-on position. Under these conditions, the hearing aid is likely to be saturated. Saturation is a characteristic of all amplifiers, and the hearing aid is no exception. The amplifier is simply incapable of producing output exceeding a certain value, known as the saturation level.

The gain and SSPL of a hearing aid are interrelated. This notion is illustrated in Figure 7.4. The function shown in this figure is known as an input-output function because it displays the output along the ordinate as a function of the input level along the abscissa. For this hypothetical input-output function, the volume control is assumed to be in the full-on position. Note that low input levels (50–60 dB SPL) reveal output values that exceed the input by 25 dB. That is, the gain (output minus input) is 25 dB at low input levels. At high input levels (90–100 dB SPL), on the other hand, the output remains constant at 110 dB SPL. This is the saturation sound pressure level of the hearing aid. The instrument simply can't produce an output higher than 110 dB SPL. Because the hearing aid is saturated, the gain at these higher input levels is lower. The gain for the 90- and 100-dB inputs is 20 and 10 dB, respectively. Because of this interaction between gain and SSPL, gain is usually measured for input levels of 50–60 dB. These are also levels that approximate those of conversational speech, the input signal of greatest interest.

Candidacy For Amplification

How does one know whether an individual is a good candidate for amplification? We have already indicated that the ideal candidate for amplification is one who displays a sensorineural hearing loss. Many audiologists use the degree of hearing loss as a "rule of thumb" for determining hearing aid candidacy. A general guideline based on the average (500–2000 Hz) pure-tone hearing loss in the better ear is summarized in Figure 7.5. As hearing loss increases, the need for assistance increases, reaching a maximum for moderate amounts of hearing loss. Potential benefit from amplification, however, is lowest at the two extremes, mild and profound impairment. Those individuals with the mildest hearing losses and those with the most profound hearing deficits are usually the candidates who will benefit the least from a hearing aid. There are many exceptions to this pure-tone-based "rule of thumb." Because of this, there is now a tendency to move away from these pure-tone guidelines and to consider anyone with a communicative difficulty as the result of hearing impairment a candidate for amplification.

There are other considerations in determining hearing aid candidacy. Some of these factors include the patient's motivation for seeking assistance, the patient's acceptance of the hearing loss, and the patient's cosmetic concerns. Even if a significant hearing loss is present, some patients put off seeking assistance for several years. The reasons for this delay are not altogether clear, although the cost of the hearing aid and the failure of the primary-care physician to refer for a hearing aid are considered contributing factors. Table 7.1 summarizes those factors that influence patients to pursue amplification. Note that communication problems at home, in noisy situations, or in social settings represent the major motivating factors for wanting a hearing aid.

Acceptance of a hearing loss is another consideration in determining hearing aid candidacy. There are some individuals who simply deny that a hearing problem exists. This is particularly true for those individuals with very mild

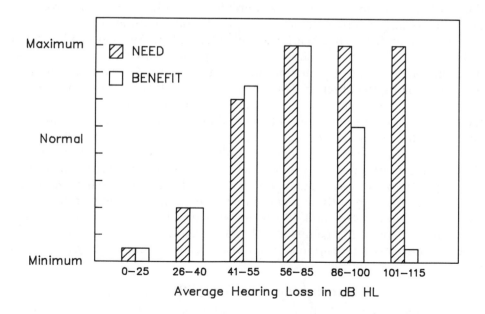

Figure 7.5. Illustration of the need for and potential benefit from amplification as a function of degree of hearing loss.

Table 7.1.
Factors That Influence a Patient's Decision to Obtain Amplification[a]

Factor	Percentage Reporting Strong or Moderate Influence
Communication problems at home	82
Communication problems in noisy listening situations	81
Communication problems in social settings	81
Communication problems at work	77
Encouragement from spouse	77

[a]Adapted from Mueller HG, Grimes A: Amplification systems for the hearing impaired. In Alpiner JG, McCarthy PA (eds): *Rehabilitative Audiology: Children and Adults.* Baltimore, Williams & Wilkins, 1987 p 119.

losses, those who fear loss of employment, and those who have suffered gradual onset of hearing loss.

Finally, one cannot overlook cosmetic concerns when considering a patient's candidacy for amplification. There continues to be a stigma associated with wearing amplification. While the acceptance of hearing aids is improving, there remains a large number of hearing-impaired individuals who are concerned about the stigma associated with amplification, especially the more conspicuous instruments. (body and BTE aids)

Hearing Aid Selection and Evaluation

Once it has been established that an individual can benefit from amplification, an appointment for hearing aid selection and evaluation is usually scheduled. In the selection phase, some important clinical decisions must be made. For example, what type of hearing aid would be most appropriate for a given hearing-impaired person? Recall from Figure 7.1 that there are a number of different types of hearing aids available in the marketplace. The audiologist needs to decide whether the patient will benefit most from a body-type hearing aid, a BTE instrument, or one of the in-the-ear systems (ITE or ITC). As noted earlier, most hearing aids sold today are BTE, ITE, or ITC units. BTE hearing aids have several distinct advantages over body aids, the most important of which are cosmetic appeal, improved sound localization, and better speech understanding in noise when two aids are worn. Importantly, very few young children wear ITE or ITC systems because of the frequent need to recast the earpiece due to a growing ear canal. Currently, about 75% of hearing aids selected for children are BTE systems. Sometimes it is appropriate to use a hearing aid that includes a bone conduction transducer. Bone conduction hearing aids are used most often in patients with pinna deformities such as those discussed in Chapter 5.

Another important clinical decision that must be made in the selection phase is whether to recommend one hearing aid (monaural amplification) or two hearing aids (binaural amplification). For years, there has been considerable controversy over the true benefits of binaural amplification. While one would intuitively think that binaural amplification is superior to monaural amplification, it has traditionally been difficult to demonstrate any objective advantages for two hearing aids. More recently, however, there has been mounting evidence in favor of binaural fittings. Based on research in this area, some of the reported advantages to binaural amplification include better sound localization, binaural summation (a sound is easier to hear with two ears than with one), and improvement in speech recognition in noise. Experienced hearing aid users often favor binaural amplification and report that two aids offer more balanced hearing, better overall hearing, improved speech clarity in noise, improved sound localization skills, and more natural and less stressful listening. Accordingly, binaural amplification has been recommended with increased regularity during the past several years. There are several other decisions that must be considered in the selection process but are beyond the scope of an introductory text. Briefly, the audiologist must consider the type of microphone (directional versus omnidirectional), earmold material (soft silastic versus hard acrylic), and type of earmold.

Modern-day hearing aids provide a wide range of electroacoustic characteristics that can be selected on the basis of the patient's individual needs. The process of selecting a hearing aid with the appropriate electroacoustic characteristics for a particular patient is referred to as hearing aid selection. This process has undergone major changes in recent years. Today most audiologists use a prescriptive approach to hearing aid selection. Using information obtained from the patient, such as the pure-tone thresholds, the appropriate gain can be prescribed according to some underlying theoretical principles. From the mid-1970s through the mid-1980s, at least a dozen different prescriptive hearing aid selection methods were developed. Although they differ in detail, these methods have the same general feature that more gain is prescribed at those frequencies for which the hearing loss is greatest. As an example, one of the simplest approaches makes use of the so-called "half-gain rule." One simply measures the hearing threshold at several frequencies and multiplies the hearing loss by a factor of one-half. Thus, for a patient with a flat 50-dB hearing loss from 250 through 8000 Hz, the appropriate gain would be 25 dB (0.5×50 dB) at each frequency. A person having a sloping hearing loss with a 40-dB HL hearing threshold at 1000 Hz and an 80-dB HL threshold at 4000 Hz would require gain of 20 and 40 dB, respectively, using this simple one-half gain rule. Regardless of the prescriptive method used, once the prescription is made, the audiologist searches among existing hearing aids to find the hearing aid with the most appropriate gain characteristics. For ITE and ITC hearing aids, the instrument is simply ordered using the prescribed gain values.

Saturation sound pressure level (SSPL) can also be prescribed for the patient. Usually additional information is required from the patient. One common approach is to measure the loudness discomfort level (LDL) of the patient for tones or narrow bands of noise. The LDL is a measure of the maximum sound level that the patient can tolerate at each frequency. It would not be desirable for the hearing aid's acoustic output to exceed the maximum tolerable level of the patient because this might cause the patient to reject the hearing aid. The SSPL of the hearing aid is frequently adjusted to a value slightly lower than the LDL. In this way, the audiologist can be assured that the acoustic output of the hearing aid will not exceed the maximum tolerance level of the patient.

Once the appropriate prescription has been made and the hearing aid(s) selected, the next process, the hearing aid evaluation, is conducted. Again, just as in the prescriptive process, there are several alternative hearing aid evaluation procedures from which the audiologist can choose. These alternatives, however, have a common goal: evaluation of the benefit provided by the hearing aid when it is worn by the hearing-impaired patient. In that the primary benefit to be derived from use of the hearing aid is improved understanding of speech, the hearing aid evaluation usually involves the measurement of the patient's speech-recognition performance with and without the hearing aid. This is done using loudspeakers with the patient positioned in the sound field. Standardized tape-recorded speech materials are preferred for testing. (See Chapter 4.) The patient is typically presented with a sample of continuous speech or speech-shaped noise at a level approximating conversational levels (65 or 70 dB SPL).

While listening to this stimulus, the patient adjusts the volume control on the hearing aid to a comfortable setting. Next, speech-recognition testing is conducted, with the materials being presented at the same overall level (65–70 dB SPL). Speech-recognition testing is often performed both in quiet and in a background of noise or multitalker babble. This is done to permit evaluation of the benefit provided by the hearing aid for a range of conditions representative of those in which the hearing aid is to be worn. With this in mind, a speech-to-noise or speech-to-babble ratio of +6–8 dB is recommended for use. This range of values is representative of "typical" noisy conditions encountered by most patients. The speech-recognition measures are also obtained in quiet and in noise under identical stimulus conditions without the hearing aid being worn by the patient. The difference in performance between the aided and unaided measures provides a general indication of the benefit provided by the hearing aid under various listening conditions.

Hearing Aid Orientation

Once the hearing aid has been selected and evaluated, the patient is counseled about the measured benefits, the limitations of hearing aids, the cost of the instrument(s), and so forth. If the patient decides to purchase the hearing aid, the audiologist may either dispense the hearing aid or refer the patient to another party who sells the recommended hearing aid. As noted in Chapter 1, an increasing percentage of audiologists today are directly involved in the dispensing of hearing aids. Hearing aids are sold on a 30-day trial basis with refunds provided for dissatisfied patients at the end of that trial period. During the trial period, the patient is encouraged to visit the audiologist two or three times for a series of hearing aid orientations. During the hearing aid orientations, the patient is instructed in the use and care of the hearing aid, counseled about its limitations and strategies to use to maximize its benefit, and given an opportunity to voice any complaints about its function. Frequently, the earmold or the earpiece of the ITE will need some modification to make the hearing aid fit more comfortably in the patient's ear. After the 30-day trial period, the hearing aid user is encouraged to return for further evaluation in a year, or sooner if experiencing difficulty.

Alternative Rehabilitative Devices

Assistive Listening Devices

As mentioned previously, full-time use of a hearing aid is not necessary or beneficial for many hearing-impaired individuals. Many people with mild hearing loss require only part-time use of a hearing aid or alternative device. For many of these individuals, a practical alternative is a class of devices known as assistive listening devices. These devices are typically electroacoustic devices designed with a much more limited purpose in mind than the conventional hearing aid. Two of the most common purposes for which these devices were developed are use of the telephone and listening to the television. Several telephone handsets have been developed, for instance, that can amplify the telephone signal by 15–30 dB. These devices are effective for people with mild hearing loss who have difficulty communicating over the telephone.

Many of the assistive listening devices physically separate the microphone from the rest of the device so that the microphone can be placed closer to the source of the desired sound. Recall that the microphone converts an acoustic signal into an electrical one so that it can be amplified by the device. If the microphone on the assistive listening device is separated by a great distance from the rest of the device, the electrical signal from the microphone must somehow be sent to the amplifier. This is accomplished in various ways, with some devices simply running a wire, several feet in length, directly from the microphone to the amplifier. Other devices convert the electrical signal from the microphone into radio waves (FM) or invisible light waves (infrared) and send the signal to a receiver adjacent to the amplifier and worn by the individual. The receiver converts the FM or infrared signal back to an electrical signal and sends it to the amplifier to be amplified. The FM and infrared systems are frequently referred to as wireless systems because they eliminate the long wire running directly from the microphone to the amplifier. The wireless feature of these assistive listening devices makes them more versatile and easier to use, but it also makes them more expensive. These assistive listening devices overcome the primary disadvantage of the conventional hearing aid; they improve the speech-to-noise ratio. By separating the microphone from the rest of the device and positioning it closer to the sound source (e.g., the talker's mouth or the loudspeaker of the television set), the primary signal of interest is amplified more than the surrounding background noise. On a conventional hearing aid, the ear-level microphone amplifies both the speech and the surrounding noise equally well. That is, the speech-to-noise ratio is not improved; all sound at the position of the microphone is simply made louder by the conventional hearing aid.

Separating the microphone from the rest of the device, however, has its drawbacks. It is only a reasonable alternative when the sound source is fairly stable over time. If the microphone is positioned near the loudspeaker of the television, for example, no amplification will be provided for the voice of a talker seated next to the impaired person. The impaired individual is forced to listen to the sound source closest to the microphone. For assistive listening devices, this is not a serious drawback because they are intended for a limited purpose.

Selection and evaluation of assistive listening devices is not as formalized as it is for hearing aids. Most clinics today have a room designated as the "assistive listening device area." This room or area is set up to simulate the conditions under which the devices are to be used. Typically, the room takes on the atmosphere of a living room or family room, with television, stereo, and telephones available. After the patient's needs have been assessed through a written or oral questionnaire, several assistive devices are tried by the patient in the simulated environment under controlled conditions. If the patient finds the device beneficial, it is dispensed by the audiologist, or the patient is referred to an appropriate source for its purchase.

Assistive devices of various types are also beneficial to the severely or profoundly impaired. In addition to those devices mentioned above, some non-auditory devices have been developed. Devices have been produced that flash lights in response to various acoustic signals occurring in the home, such as the ringing of the doorbell or the telephone. Other special telephone devices enable text to be sent over phone lines (in printed form) so that a profoundly impaired person can carry on a telephone conversation by sending and receiving text messages. Special keyboard-like devices are needed at both ends of the phone line to enable such communication.

Classroom Amplification

A discussion of hearing aids would not be complete without a review of the special amplification systems designed for education. Classroom amplification is a term used to describe a hearing aid device that provides amplified sound to a group of children. Classroom amplification gained added importance with the advent of Public Law 94–142, a federal mandate regarding the education of all handicapped children. The law required that schools provide hearing-impaired children with adequate services and funding. This included habilitative/rehabilitative services such as selection and evaluation of personal hearing aids and group systems, auditory training, speech training, speechreading and any other services deemed necessary for the child's educational development.

Why should a child need a special educational amplification system? A primary concern is the acoustic environment that children are exposed to in the classroom. Children are continually bombarded with excessively high noise levels that interfere with their ability to understand the teacher. These noise levels originate from sources outside the school building (aircraft, car traffic), within the school building (adjacent classrooms and hallways, activity areas, heating/cooling systems), and from within the classroom itself (students talking, feet shuffling, noise from moving furniture). These various noise sources contribute to noise levels ranging from 40 to 67 dB SPL (A).[a] Such high noise levels result in an unfavorable signal-to-noise (S:N) or speech-to-noise ratio reaching the child's ear. Recall that a S:N ratio represents the difference in dB between speech (the teacher) and the overall ambient noise (within the classroom). For example, a S:N ratio of +10 means that the teacher's speech is 10 dB more intense than the noise in the classroom. Ideally, a S:N ratio of +20 dB is necessary if a hearing-impaired child is to understand speech maximally. Noise surveys in classrooms have shown that S:N ratios typically range from −6 dB to +6 dB, a listening environment that precludes maximal understanding even for normal-hearing children.

---

[a] Sound level meters have three weighting networks: A, B, and C, which are designed to respond differently to the frequencies of noise. The A network weighs (filters) the low frequencies and approximates the response characteristics of the human ear. The B network also filters the low frequencies, but not as much as the A network. The C scale provides a fairly flat response. The federal government recommends the use of the A network for measuring noise levels.

Classroom noise is not the only variable that contributes to a difficult listening environment. Reverberation, a term used to denote the amount of time it takes for sound to decrease by 60 dB following the termination of a signal, also contributes to an adverse acoustic environment. When a teacher talks to the child, some of the speech signal reaches the child's amplification system within just a few milliseconds. The remainder of the signal, however, strikes surrounding areas and reaches the child's ear a few milliseconds after the initial sound in the form of reflections. The strength and duration of these reflections are affected by the absorption quality of the surrounding surfaces and the size (volume) of the classroom. If an area has hard walls, ceilings, and floors, the room will have a long reverberation time. In contrast, an acoustically treated room with carpeting, drapes, and an acoustic tile ceiling will have a shorter reverberation time. Generally, as reverberation time increases, speech recognition decreases. In addition, the smaller the room size, the greater the reverberation. Many classrooms for the hearing impaired have reverberation times ranging from a very mild value of 0.02 seconds to more severe reverberation, with times greater than 1 second.

These factors, noise and reverberation, are known to produce an adverse effect on speech recognition. As the noise levels and reverberation times increase, the S:N ratio becomes less favorable and there is a significant breakdown in speech understanding. Further, as the distance between the talker and listener increases, the S:N ratio worsens. An example of this phenomenon is shown in Figure 7.6. This figure illustrates the speech-recognition scores for sentence materials in a group of normal-hearing children who listened to speech with noise levels and reverberation times similar to those in a classroom. The reverberation time is 0.46 second, and the S:N ratio at 6 feet is +6 dB. Note that speech recognition deteriorates with increasing distance. At 6 feet, speech recognition is seen to average about 90%, while at 24 feet, it averages 40%. An example of how noise and reverberation can produce a hardship for young hearing-impaired children is shown in Table 7.2. These data represent the unaided speech-recogni-

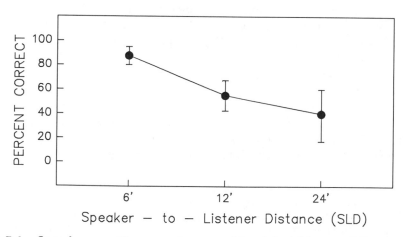

Figure 7.6.   Speech recognition score for normal-hearing children at different speaker-to-listener distances. At 6 feet the S:N ratio is +6 dB and the reverberation time is 0.46 sec.

Table 7.2.
Mean Word Recognition Scores for Hearing-Impaired Children with Hearing Aids under Various Noise and Reverberant Conditions[a]

Reverberation Time (seconds)	Signal-to-Noise Ratio (dB)			
	Quiet	+12	+6	0
0.0 (nonreverberant)	83	70	60	39
0.4	74	60	52	28
1.2	45	41	27	11

[a]Adapted from Finitzo-Hieber T, Tillman TW: Room acoustic effects on monosyllabic word discrimination ability for normal and hearing impaired children. *J Speech Hear Res* 21:440–448, 1978.

tion scores of hearing-impaired children in quiet, and under different S:N ratios and reverberation times. It is seen that as the noise levels increase, speech recognition decreases. Further, as reverberation increases, speech recognition decreases. At an S:N ratio of +6 dB (a common listening condition in the classroom) with a reverberation time of 0.4 second, the mean recognition score is 52%; when reverberation time is 1.2 seconds, recognition is only 27%. It is not surprising that a hearing-impaired child will experience considerable difficulty trying to learn under such adverse conditions.

Several types of special educational amplification systems have been designed to overcome the adverse effects of the classroom environment by offering a better S:N ratio. These system types include hard-wire systems, FM wireless systems, infrared systems, and a system that combines the FM wireless system with a personal hearing aid. The concept behind these systems is similar to that described for the assistive listening devices. The microphone is moved closer to the desired sound source, the teacher. A brief description of each of these systems follows.

Hard-wire System

In this system, a microphone worn by the teacher is wired to an amplifier. Each student then wears headphones or insert-type receivers that are connected to the amplifier by wires, so that the teacher and the students are, in effect, "tethered" together (Fig. 7.7**A**). The primary advantage of a hard-wire system is the high fidelity and high level of output available through earphones. These systems are inexpensive and are simple and easy to operate. The obvious disadvantage is the restricted mobility of both the teacher and students.

FM Wireless Systems

About 65% of all classrooms for the hearing impaired use either FM devices or a combination of an FM system and a personal hearing aid. A microphone transmitter is worn around the teacher's neck, and a signal is broadcast to an FM receiver worn by the child. Most FM receivers have an environmental microphone so that the child can monitor his or her own voice, the voices of his or her peers, and other environmental sounds (Fig. 7.7**B**). When the environmental

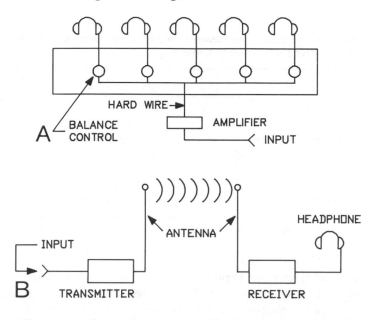

Figure 7.7. Illustration of two classroom amplification systems. **A**, hard-wire; **B**, FM. The personal hearing aid could replace the headphones shown in **B** to produce a dovetail system.

microphone is used, however, the S:N ratio is compromised because of the distance between the talker and the microphone. The advantage to this system is the mobility allowed. In other words, the teacher and the students are free to move around the room and the students will continue to receive amplification.

Infrared Systems

Infrared group amplification is seldom used in classroom settings but is in widespread use as an assistive device in theaters, churches, and other public facilities. As mentioned earlier, the system employs an infrared emitter that transmits the speech signal from the input microphone to individually worn infrared-receiver/audio-amplifier units. These systems are somewhat limited in power output.

Combining the FM Wireless System with the Personal Hearing Aid

A number of attempts have been made to combine the personal hearing aid with the FM system. This approach, commonly referred to as dovetailing, is done to take advantage of the benefits of both systems; the improved speech-to-noise ratio offered by the FM system and the custom fitting of the personal hearing aid. A commonly accepted method for combining the FM system with the personal hearing aid is the use of an electrical connection from the student-worn receiver to the child's hearing aid amplifier. Most modern-day BTE aids can be designed to accept an electrical plug from the student's FM receiver unit. This combined system has the capability for FM input alone, FM input plus the signal from the microphone of the personal hearing aid, and input from the microphone of the personal hearing aid alone.

Cochlear Implants

A relatively recent clinical development has been the emergence of the cochlear implant as a alternative to conventional amplification. There are several types of cochlear implants available commercially today. They all share a common conceptual framework but differ in how it is implemented in each device. The cochlear implant is a device that is surgically implanted with its stimulating electrodes (wires) inserted directly into the cochlea. The implant contains from one to 22 electrodes. The electrodes are used to stimulate the auditory nerve directly with electric current, bypassing the damaged cochlear structures. As in the conventional hearing aid, a microphone is used to convert the acoustic signal into an electrical one. The electrical signal is then amplified and processed in various ways in a separate, body-worn component known as the stimulator. The stimulator is about the size of a body-worn hearing aid or a package of cigarettes. The output of the stimulator is then sent to an electromagnetic receiver worn behind the ear. This external receiver generates a magnetic field which, in turn, activates a similar internal receiver implanted surgically just under the skin and behind the ear. The implanted internal receiver converts the magnetic signal into an electrical one and directs it to the electrode(s) penetrating the cochlea. This electrical signal, when routed to the electrodes, stimulates the remaining healthy auditory nerve fibers of the damaged inner ear. Figure 7.8 illustrates a typical arrangement for a single-electrode cochlear implant and compares this device to a conventional hearing aid. As can be seen, many common features are shared by these two devices.

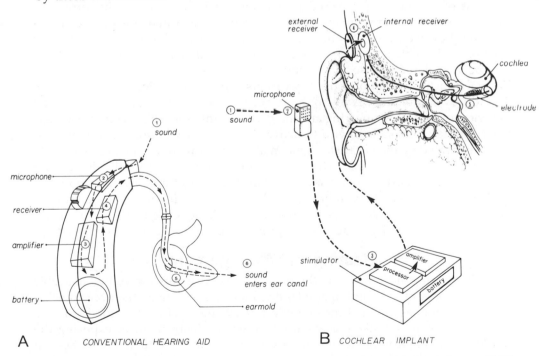

Figure 7.8. Illustration of the similarities between **A**, conventional behind-the-ear (BTE) hearing aid and **B**, cochlear implant device. The components of each system are numbered identically to highlight the similarities.

At present, the ideal candidates for cochlear implants are persons who have profound bilateral sensorineural hearing loss and have acquired the hearing loss after the acquisition of language. Although the results of clinical trials with these devices have varied markedly between patients, the best performance appears to be achieved with the multi-electrode devices. There are examples of so-called "star" patients who perform remarkably well with the device by itself; however, the majority of people fitted thus far appear to derive the greatest benefit from the device when it is used as an aid to speechreading. Its primary usefulness as an aid to speechreading appears to lie in making gross cues of timing and voicing available to the patient. At a minimum, the cochlear implants appear to provide an awareness of sound to the once-silent world of the deafened patient. At its present stage of development, however, the cochlear implant is an alternative for only a very small percentage of the hearing-impaired population: those without usable residual hearing sensitivity.

Vibrotactile Devices

For many profoundly hearing-impaired persons, little or no meaningful information can be conveyed through the auditory sensory modality. This is true whether the auditory modality is stimulated with an acoustic signal in the case of the conventional hearing aid or an electrical one in the case of the cochlear implant. Often this results in the use of alternative means of communication using normally functioning sensory modalities. Manual communication, or sign language, takes advantage of the normally functioning visual modality that exists in most of the hearing-impaired population, including those with profound impairments. Adoption of manual communication as a primary means of communicating, however, restricts one to communicating with the small percentage of the population able to converse in sign language. Other sensory modalities have also been explored for use as alternative means of encoding the acoustic signal. Tactual (touch) stimulation is used by various vibrotactile devices as an alternative to auditory stimulation. A microphone again converts the acoustic signal to an electrical one, as in the hearing aid and cochlear implant. This electrical signal is used by the vibrotactile device to activate a series of vibrators. The vibrators, when activated by the electrical signal, make contact with the skin and stimulate the patient's sense of touch. The most common clinical vibrotactile devices are single-channel instruments. They stimulate the skin at a constant rate or frequency and increase the amplitude of vibration as the intensity of the acoustic signal increases. The vibrators for most clinical devices are worn on the hand, wrist, arm, or thigh. These devices are primarily used as an aid to speechreading.

Hearing Aid Management

The hearing aid represents the most important rehabilitative tool available for the majority of hearing-impaired individuals. It is essential that every precaution be taken to assure that the amplification system is always in good working order. Care must be taken to avoid dropping the instrument or exposing the aid to severe environmental conditions, such as excessive moisture or heat. If dampness reaches the microphone or receiver, it can render the unit inoperable. It is also important to check the earmold or canal portion of the device periodically for blockage by cerumen and signs of wear from extended use, such as a cracked earmold or tubing. Perhaps the most common problem that interferes with adequate hearing aid performance is the battery or battery compartment area. Old batteries that have lost their charge, inappropriate battery size, inadequate battery contact, and improper battery placement are all problems that can contribute to a nonworking hearing aid.

Consistent amplification for the young hearing-impaired child is essential. Yet numerous school surveys have revealed that about one-half of children's hearing aids do not perform satisfactorily. The most common problems seen among hearing-impaired children are weak batteries, inadequate earmolds, broken cords, bad receivers (sometimes wrong receiver), and high distortion levels. Even the FM-wireless systems are susceptible to faulty performance. About 30–50% of these systems have been reported to perform unsatisfactorily in the classroom setting. The solution to inconsistent and inadequate amplification is the implementation of a daily hearing-aid check using a form similar to that shown in Vignette 7.1. In addition, the school audiologist must conduct a periodic electroacoustic analysis of every child's hearing aid.

REHABILITATION OF THE HEARING-IMPAIRED CHILD

Management of the hearing-impaired child represents a monumental challenge to the clinical audiologist. In learning to understand the spoken language of others and to speak it, there is no adequate substitute for an intact auditory system. Without normal or near-normal hearing, it is extremely difficult to acquire an adequate communication system. Because so much of the language-learning process occurs within the first few years of life, there has been considerable emphasis on early identification and intervention for young hearing-impaired children. The various approaches to early identification have been outlined in Chapter 6 and will not be restated here. Suffice it to say that it is generally believed that the earlier one can identify the hearing loss, preferably during the 1st year of life, the sooner intervention can begin and the better the chances for a favorable outcome. Generally speaking, those hearing impaired children who exhibit the best spoken language and show the most satisfactory progress in school are those who have had the benefit of early identification and intervention. Early intervention is essential to the successful development of speech and language. The intervention must include adequate parent-infant management, wearable amplification, speech and language training, and development of perceptual and cognitive skills.

Choosing the Appropriate Communication Mode

An important issue facing audiologists, teachers, and school officials is determining which educational approach is most appropriate for a given hearing-impaired child. Presently, there exist two primary modes of instruction recommended in the educational system: auditory-oral communication and total communication. The auditory-oral approach places emphasis entirely on the auditory system for developing receptive and expressive forms of communication, whereas total communication emphasizes a combination of audition, vision, finger spelling and signs for achieving the same goal. These approaches will be discussed in greater detail in Chapter 8. Although most would agree that oral language is desirable in order to maximize the options available to the child, the

---

Vignette 7.1.   Sample Monitoring Form for a Personal Hearing Aid Worn by a Hearing-Impaired Child

Student_____

Teacher_____ Aid make/model_____

School_____ Serial no. _____

Classroom_____

Electroacoustic check   ___Y ___N

Date of inspection_____

Overall condition: ___Satisfactory ___Marginal ___Unsatisfactory ___Missing

Recommendations_____

_____

_____

Examiner_____

Problem Checklist

Item	Inspected?: Yes	No	Comments
Battery	___	___	_____
Battery compartment	___	___	_____
Microphone	___	___	_____
Power switch	___	___	_____
Gain control	___	___	_____
Telephone switch	___	___	_____
Tone control	___	___	_____
Amplifier	___	___	_____
Cord	___	___	_____
Receiver	___	___	_____
Earmold	___	___	_____
Clip/case	___	___	_____
Harness	___	___	_____
Other	___	___	_____

As-worn setting:
   Volume control_____
   Tone control_____
   Receiver type_____

---

reality is that not all children are able to learn spoken English. Even in total communication programs, decisions are sometimes made about whether to emphasize oral language or manual communication. How then does one determine which mode of communication is most beneficial?

Two approaches have been proposed for determining whether a hearing-impaired child would be better off in an auditory-oral or a total-communication program of instruction. The Deafness Management Quotient (DMQ) has been developed. The DMQ uses a weighted point system (total of 100 points) to quantify a number of factors about the child and the child's environment. These factors include the amount of residual hearing (30 points), central auditory system intactness (30 points), intellectual factors (20 points), family constellation (10 points), and socioeconomic issues (10 points). A child scoring greater than 80 points would be recommended for an auditory-oral program. Unfortunately, it is very difficult to quantify objectively the recommended factors, and more importantly, the DMQ has not undergone adequate validation. More recently, an alternative index known as the Spoken Language Predictor (SLP) has been proposed and validated. Similar to the DMQ, the SLP incorporates five factors considered important to a child's success in an auditory-oral program. The factors are weighted, and a point score (total of 100 points) is derived. The factors include hearing capacity (30 points), language competence (25 points), nonverbal intelligence (20 points), family support (15 points), and speech-communication attitude (10 points). Children with scores of 80–100 are judged to have excellent potential for developing spoken language. Not only can the SLP be of use in deciding on placement, but it can also verify the appropriateness of placement for an older child already enrolled in a program.

Let us now review some of the appropriate management strategies for hearing-impaired children. The approaches to be discussed can accommodate either an auditory-oral or a total communication emphasis.

Parent-Infant Management

It is recognized that the first 3 years of life are critical to the child's general development, especially with respect to communication. It is also recognized that the parents of young handicapped children often lack the skills necessary to optimize family-infant interactions, which could facilitate the child's communication development. From this awareness, parent-infant intervention programs have emerged. In addition to espousing early identification and intervention, most parent-oriented programs include family support for parents and members of the child's extended family. Information sharing or exchange, demonstration teaching in which the family explores a variety of strategies to assist their child in achieving communication, and educational advocacy for the parents are also frequently included. The latter entails helping the parents to become effective consumers of services and knowledgeable child advocates.

An important component of a parent-infant curriculum is audiologic management and amplification. Here the emphasis is on helping the child to develop his/her auditory potential. Emphasis is placed on further clarification of the nature of the hearing loss, selection of amplification, and the development of full-time hearing aid use. Teaching parents the importance of care and maintenance of hearing aids is also an important dimension. Another element of effective parent-infant management is auditory training—that is, an organized sequential approach to the development of listening skills. Here the emphasis is on developing a program of auditory training experiences that will guide the parents through a developmental sequence for their child that parallels the development of auditory perceptual skills in the normal-hearing infant. The hierarchy of skills can be divided into the following levels:

1. Auditory perception of both environmental sounds and the human voice;
2. Awareness of environmental sounds and the human voice as conveyors of information and association of sounds with their physical sources;

3. Development of an auditory-vocal feedback mechanism in which the child monitors his or her own speech;
4. Comprehension of meaning in syllables, words, phrases, and sentences;
5. Increasing verbal comprehension and the emergence of auditory memory and sequencing skills.

Another important component of parent-infant management is vocal play strategies for speech habilitation. The initiation and maintenance of vocal behavior is another major area of the early-intervention program that is critical to young children. Full-time use of amplification is important so that the hearing-impaired child can hear his or her own speech as well as the speech of others. The use of an auditory program to enhance the use of the auditory feedback mechanism is also important. Further, parents are taught to use vocal play interaction techniques that are necessary for the development of prelinguistic speech skills. Parents must also learn to develop strategies that facilitate social and communicative turn-taking.

Finally, there are the verbal interaction techniques of language programming. At this point the focus is on teaching the parent communicative interaction styles, particularly verbal interaction patterns, that enhance the child's acquisition of language. Linguistic development is maximized by training parents to incorporate those principles of adult-child interaction patterns that are reported to occur during the language acquisition of normal children.

Amplification

The importance of amplification to the hearing-impaired child cannot be overemphasized. The personal hearing aid and other amplification devices represent the primary link many of these children have to an auditory society. If these children are to develop speech and language in a manner somewhat similar to the normal-hearing child, everything possible must be done to capitalize on whatever residual hearing exists. Toward this end, the child receives amplification (usually binaural) soon after identification. The audiologist then offers periodic hearing evaluations and modifies the hearing aid fitting(s) as more is learned about the child's hearing sensitivity.

Language: Characteristics, Assessment, and Training

Language may be defined as a set of systematic rules used to designate experience and facilitate social interaction. It is the primary means by which humans communicate with one another. Although a comprehensive review of language is beyond the scope of this book, a general knowledge of the dimensions of language is important to the understanding of management issues. Most would agree that there are three components of language: form, content, and use. The form of language is simply the pattern of sounds, syllables, words, and sentences that are used to express thoughts and ideas. For example, the endings /t/ and /d/ in "talk*ed*" and "pray*ed*" both express past tense, yet the phonetic forms of the past-tense morphemes (a morpheme is the smallest grammatical unit of language) are quite different. To learn language, children must possess the capacity to identify and process such subtle nuances. Form can be further categorized into phonology, morphology, and syntax. Phonology is the sound system of a given language. Morphology is concerned with the structure of words (i.e., plurals, possessives). Syntax addresses the relationship of words with larger units of language, such as phrases, clauses, and sentences. The second aspect of language is content, or what is being communicated. This is often referred to as the semantic level of language. The content is concerned with the knowledge of objects, the knowledge of relationships between or among objects, and the knowledge of relationships among other things. The final component of language is use, which represents how one communicates. This has been referred to as pragmatics. It is learning to transmit information appropriately and intentionally. It is achieving a goal set about by communicating. For example, a child can point to a cookie and say "more," indicating communicative intent. Hence, the pragmatic component of language is present in the absence of syntax. The development of language is a complex interaction that occurs among these three components of language: form, content, and use.

Given what we have discussed about language, it is not surprising to learn that children with hearing loss experience great difficulty in learning language through the speech modality. This difficulty increases with increasing hearing loss. Most research dealing with the language characteristics of hearing-impaired children has focused on the "form" component, primarily because errors in form (phonemes, morphemes, and syntax) are easier to quantify. Studies have shown that hearing-impaired children with high-frequency hearing losses experience difficulty with morphologic markers, such as plurals and possessives. In addition, it is well recognized that hearing-impaired children have trouble learning vocabulary, acquiring words that express relationships between other words, and learning syntactic structures.

There are many commercially available instruments designed to assist the clinician in the ongoing evaluation of a child's language development. These evaluative approaches explore a wide range of language skills but, for the most part, do not cover some of the experiences encountered in day-to-day situations. Hence, clinicians always need to develop informal nonstandardized tasks to obtain information in areas not covered by the standard diagnostic tools.

Historically, there have been a number of approaches used in language intervention, most of which have focused on the syntactic forms of language. These approaches can be classified as analytic or natural methods for teaching language. Analytic methods have concentrated on the form of a child's language, and most techniques are involved in categorizing the various parts of speech grammatically. These approaches are also characterized by extensive drills and exercises. An example of the analytical method is the Fitzgerald key, which emphasizes the analysis of relationships among discrete units through the visual aid of written language. Students classify words from a sentence as to whether they belong in a "who," "what," or "where" category. The natural approach, sometimes referred to as the experiential method, holds that language is learned through experiences, not systematic drills and exercises. This content/unit approach emphasizes identifying areas of interest for the child, which then serve as the basis for teaching vocabulary and practicing spoken and written language.

More recently, language-intervention approaches have begun to take into consideration modern language theory and to develop strategies that attempt to integrate syntactic, pragmatic, and semantic levels. The reader interested in learning more about language intervention techniques with the hearing impaired can consult the suggested readings at the end of this chapter.

Speech Production: Characteristics, Assessment, and Training

We have noted earlier that significant hearing losses result in difficulty not only in understanding speech but also in producing speech. Nevertheless, it is the general consensus that many hearing-impaired children, even those with profound losses, can develop speech skills. Hearing-impaired children manifest a variety of speech production errors categorized as either segmental (i.e., phonemic) or nonsegmental (i.e., intonation and prosody). The most common segmental errors include the omission of word-final sounds and substitution errors for both consonants and vowels. Nonsegmental errors include inadequate timing, which results in very slow, labored speech, and poor control of the fundamental frequency, causing abnormal pitch and distorted intonation. Predictably, as the frequency of errors increases, overall intelligibility decreases.

Assessment of speech production is not as easy as one might predict, since many of the tools were designed for normal-hearing children. The evaluation of segmental errors is usually conducted with commonly available picture identification tests. Since most of these tests do not take into consideration many of the problems unavoidable when testing the hearing impaired, it is not unusual for the clinician to develop informal tests that will focus on specific segmental errors frequently seen among the hearing-impaired population. Assessment of intelligibility of speech is also important for the planning of an intervention program. Some clinicians record spontaneous language samples, which are then judged by a group of listeners to evaluate a child's intelligibility.

Perhaps the most popular method for teaching speech to the hearing impaired child is an approach advocated by Daniel Ling. Very briefly, this method focuses on using the child's residual hearing to monitor speech production, as well as to understand the speech of others. The approach to speech acquisition attempts to duplicate the process that normal-hearing children experience. The teaching of speech is carried out primarily at the phonetic and phonologic levels, with emphasis on the phonetic domain. At the phonetic level, there is emphasis on nonsense syllable drills (i.e., /ta,ta,ta/, or /ti,ta,to/). Several stages are proposed in which target behaviors are established using criterion-referenced skills. A child must complete each phase satisfactorily before moving on to the next level. These stages include undifferentiated vocalizations; nonsegmental voice patterns; a range of distinctly different vowel sounds; consonants contrasted in manner of production; consonants contrasted in manner and place of production; consonants contrasted in manner, place, and voicing; and consonant blends. The following additional strategies have been suggested to supplement the Ling approach.

1. Production on an imitative basis—the child produces the target sound using auditory clues only;
2. Production on demand—the child produces the target sound from visual cues;

3. Discrimination—the child selects the speech pattern from a closed set of alternative speech patterns;
4. Self-evaluation—the child evaluates his or her own speech production.

REHABILITATION OF THE HEARING-IMPAIRED ADULT

The rehabilitation techniques employed with the hearing-impaired adult are quite different from the approaches used with children. There are, however, similarities. The individual must receive a careful assessment to determine the nature and extent of the problem; amplification plays a major role in the rehabilitation process; and the techniques and strategies used in rehabilitation are determined by the information elicited in the assessment phase.

Issues on Assessment

In the introduction to this chapter, we talked about the importance of the assessment phase and how it is used to establish a rehabilitative program. The assessment phase typically consists of a comprehensive case history, pure-tone audiometry, speech-recognition tests, a communication-specific self-assessment questionnaire, and a measure of speechreading ability. Because we have already reviewed in some detail the basic assessment battery (case history, pure-tone audiometry, and speech recognition), we will focus here on questionnaires and speechreading skills in the planning of rehabilitation programs.

Assessment with Communication Scales

Communication scales need to be a part of every assessment approach. These scales usually assess how the hearing impairment affects everyday living— that is, the way in which the hearing deficit impacts on psychosocial, social, or vocational performance. Such information can be of value in determining the need for and probable success of amplification, irrespective of the degree of hearing loss and the specific areas in which the rehabilitation should occur. Most scales have focused on communication-specific skills. Examples of questions that could be included in such a scale are: "Do you have difficulty hearing when someone speaks in a whisper?" and "Does a hearing problem cause you difficulty when listening to TV or radio?"

The answers to such questions offer insight into those listening situations where problems exist. Once the area(s) of difficulty have been identified, possible solutions can be considered. For example, if the individual reports difficulty only when listening to a television or radio, the possibility of an assistive listening device might be considered. If, on the other hand, a patient reports difficulty in a variety of listening situations and notes a tendency to withdraw from social activities because of the hearing loss, the individual would be a good candidate for a personal hearing aid. Counseling for this patient and the patient's relatives might also be indicated. Furthermore, the audiologist may wish to develop techniques for improving speechreading and auditory training skills in those situations where listening difficulty is experienced. There are numerous communication scales available to the audiologist, and it is not possible to review all of them in an introductory book. Two commonly employed scales are the Hearing Handicap Scale (HHS) and the Hearing Performance Inventory (HPI). The HHS was designed to measure objectively the impact of hearing loss on an individual's independent living skills. There are two forms, each containing 20 items, and the test requires no more than 5 minutes to administer. Examples of typical questions are: "Can you understand if someone speaks to you in a whisper and you cannot see his face?" and "Do you hear all right when you are in a streetcar, airplane, bus or train?"

The response format to the various questions is:

_____ 1. Almost always
_____ 2. Usually
_____ 3. Sometimes
_____ 4. Rarely
_____ 5. Almost never

The HPI is a more comprehensive scale than the HHS and probes hearing-impaired patients across several dimensions rather than only one. These dimensions include speech comprehension, signal intensity, response to auditory failure, social effects of hearing loss, personal effects of hearing loss, and occupational difficulties. Examples of items on the HPI are: "You are home reading in a quiet room. Do you hear the telephone ring when it is in another room?" and "At the beginning of a conversation, do you let a stranger know that you have a hearing problem?" In this inventory, the patient is queried about a specific listening environment and responds to each item with "practically always," "frequently," "about half the time," "occasionally," or "almost never." The original version of the HPI was quite long, taking about 60 minutes to administer and score. A shortened version (about 30 minutes) is now available. The HPI affords valuable information regarding the impact of hearing loss on communication and identifies the general listening situations in which the patient experiences trouble. It is also useful as a formal performance measure that can be used at the initial assessment and to track progress during rehabilitation.

Assessment of Speechreading Skills

The ability to utilize vision as an aid to understanding spoken English is another important area of assessment. There are several tests available for assessing a patient's speech-reading or lipreading skills. One such test is the Denver Quick Test of Lipreading Ability, a group of 20 short, simple statements (Table 7.3). The test is scored in terms of percent correct, with each test item representing 5%. The test can be used to assess speechreading abilities in a vision-only mode, as well as utilizing both the vision and auditory modes combined. Performance in the visual-only mode can offer valuable diagnostic information. A low score on the Denver Test would suggest that the patient is in need of speechreading instruction—that is, instruction in paying attention to visual cues for the purpose of complementing auditory input. The use of both modes offers insight into how the patient will perform under realistic conditions and should also be helpful in determining how well the individual will perform with amplification.

Management Strategies with the Hearing-Impaired Adult

The Importance of Counseling

Counseling should represent a central focus of any management strategy for the hearing-impaired adult. In fact, the hearing-impaired should receive

Table 7.3.
Illustration of Items on the Denver Quick Test of Lipreading Ability[a]

1. Good morning.
2. How old are you?
3. I live in (state of residence).
4. I only have one dollar.
5. There is somebody at the door.
6. Is that all?
7. Where are you going?
8. Let's have a coffee break.
9. Park your car in the lot.
10. What is your address?
11. May I help you?
12. I feel fine.
13. It is time for dinner.
14. Turn right at the corner.
15. Are you ready to order?
16. Is this charge or cash?
17. What time is it?
18. I have a headache.
19. How about going out tonight?
20. Please lend me 50 cents.

[a]From Alpiner JG: Evaluation of adult communication function. In Alpiner JG, McCarthy PA (eds): *Rehabilitative Audiology: Children and Adults*. Baltimore, Williams & Wilkins, 1987.

counseling both before and after the provision of a hearing aid. Counseling is a vital part of the assessment phase, since it is during this phase that information about the patient's communication problems is determined. The first component of the counseling process is to explain to the patient, in lay terms, the nature and extent of the hearing loss. If the audiologist believes that the patient can benefit from amplification, counseling is needed to discuss with the patient the value of a hearing aid and what can be expected from it. Possible modification of the patient's motivation and attitudes may also be appropriate at this juncture. The audiologist will have information from the assessment data on the patient's feelings about wearing a hearing aid. Often the patient has no real interest in a hearing aid but is simply responding to the will of a spouse or "significant other." Others have received misleading information about hearing aids from friends or from advertisements. Some patients are concerned about whether the hearing aid will show because of the stigma commonly associated with deafness in the United States. Under such circumstances, the objective of the audiologist is to help the hearing-impaired individual realize that many of the fears or concerns about hearing loss or hearing aids are unwarranted. The individual should be counseled that the use of amplification can be beneficial in a variety of listening situations. Counseling is also sometimes appropriate for relatives and friends who have developed erroneous impressions about hearing loss and amplification. For example, a patient with a high-frequency sensorineural hearing loss will typically experience difficulty in understanding speech. Relatives and friends sometimes interpret this difficulty as a sign of senility, inattention, or even stupidity. It is helpful for the audiologist to counsel relatives and friends about the nature and extent of hearing loss as well as the psychosocial complications associated with a hearing deficit. Reviewing such information with loved ones helps them to understand better and to be more tolerant of the listening difficulties caused by a significant hearing impairment. The audiologist may also choose to offer suggestions for enhancing communication. The "significant other" can be counseled in the use of deliberate, unhurried speech, good illumination of the speaker's face, and care to insure that the lips are clearly visible.

Once the hearing aid has been purchased, or just prior to a purchase, the patient is counseled about the use and care of a hearing aid. The audiologist reviews the manipulation of the various controls, the function of the battery compartment, the trouble-shooting techniques in cases of malfunction, the proper care of the earmold, and the warranty of the hearing aid. A potential difficulty is that patients often have unrealistic expectations for a hearing aid, especially in the initial stages of use. The audiologist must take care to advise the hearing-impaired patient about the limitations of amplification and to help the individual adjust to very difficult listening situations, such as competing speech or the presence of a competing background noise. Finally, some patients will need special help in the manipulation of hearing aid controls. This is a common problem among the elderly and will be discussed in more detail later in this chapter.

Throughout the entire rehabilitation cycle, counseling is seen as a continuing process. The audiologist spends time listening, advising, and reacting to the needs and concerns of the hearing-impaired individual.

Instruction for Speechreading and Auditory Training

The two primary training aspects of aural rehabilitation for the adult are speechreading and auditory training. Speechreading refers to the ability of a person, any person, to use vision as a supplement to audition when communicating. All persons, regardless of the degree of impairment, can benefit from the use of visual cues. At one time, speechreading was referred to simply as "lipreading." The change in label to "speechreading" has come about in recognition of the fact that more than just the talker's lips provide important visual cues to understanding speech.

Speechreading should be viewed not as a replacement for auditory coding of speech but as an important supplement. Using visual information alone, most individuals can understand about 50–60% of a "spoken" message. However, there are large variations among individuals in this ability.

Acquisition of speechreading skills can take hours of training. There are two basic approaches to speechreading training: analytic and synthetic. Analytic methods begin with training on individual speech sounds and progress to words, phrases, sentences, and continuous discourse, in sequence. The synthetic approach begins training at the phrase or sentence level. The synthetic approach appears to be the one more widely used by audiologists. Training usually begins with simple, commonly encountered questions such as, "What is your name?" or "What time is it?" It then progresses to less frequently encountered statements and continuous discourse.

Auditory training refers to training the hearing-impaired individual to use his or her hearing as well as possible. The approaches pursued vary depending upon the onset of the hearing loss. Typically, a hierarchy of skills is developed at the phoneme and word level, beginning with detection of the sound or word (can the patient hear anything when the sound is spoken?). The next goal is discrimination of the targeted sound or word (is it the same or different from some other sounds or words?), and finally the identification of the sound or word (what was it?). Auditory training is encouraged for all individuals wearing a hearing aid for the first time. It takes time and training to learn to understand speech with a hearing aid. Many hearing-impaired individuals have never heard speech or have heard it through the distortion introduced by the hearing loss— in many cases, for a period of several years before seeking assistance. Fitting the hearing aid or other rehabilitative device will not bring about an instant restoration of normal function. In fact, most patients will probably never perform like a normal-hearing person. With continued training, however, they can come much closer to achieving this objective. Auditory training is designed to maximize the use of residual hearing, while speechreading is meant to supplement the reduced information received through the auditory system. Extensive training in both areas can result in very effective use of the rehabilitative device chosen for the patient.

Listening Training, Speech Conservation, and Speech Tracking

Another role of the audiologist is to help the hearing-impaired patient develop or maintain good listening skills and to assist the patient in maintaining good speech production skills. Listening training refers to helping the patient to attend better to the spoken message. Some people simply have poor listening skills, and this problem is exacerbated in the presence of a hearing loss. The emphasis in listening training is on teaching the impaired listener to be alert, attentive, and ready to receive the spoken message. Training should focus on eliminating or avoiding distractions, learning to focus on the speaker's main points, attending to nonverbal information, keeping visual contact with the speaker, and mentally preparing oneself to listen to the speaker.

As hearing loss increases, it becomes more difficult for an individual to monitor his or her own speech production. The inability to monitor the spoken message results in faulty speech characterized by poor vocal quality, nasality, segmental errors, and nonsegmental errors. Under such conditions, learning the effective use of kinesthetic cues is essential for creating an awareness of the segmental elements of speech. The patient must become physically aware of the kinesthetic (sensation of movement) qualities of each phonetic element in speech. Auditory training and speechreading can also help in preserving the perception of subtle nuances in the speech message. Techniques for developing an awareness of the rhythm, quality, intonation, and loudness of one's own speech are needed by the hearing impaired. Finally, the importance of listening is critical to this population, and the enhancement of listening skills should be part of any speech conservation program.

Speech tracking refers to a procedure in which connected speech is presented by a reader, and a listener repeats the message back word for word or syllable for syllable. Both the speaker and the listener participate in the procedure, with the impaired listener attempting to immediately imitate the speaker. The technique has great face validity since the material approximates normal communication more closely than single words. Tracking ability is measured in terms of the number of words tracked per minute. Rate of speech tracking improves with rehabilitative training (speechreading and/or auditory training) and with the use of amplification or alternative rehabilitation devices. Speech tracking can be used as a tool in aural rehabilitation, especially for measuring pre- and posttraining effects.

Special Considerations for the Hearing-Impaired Elderly

We have noted on several occasions throughout this text that a large number of elderly people exhibit significant hearing impairments. Typically, the hearing impairment in the aged is a mild-to-moderate bilateral high-frequency sensorineural hearing loss with associated difficulty in understanding conversational speech. The loss usually begins around 50 years of age and progresses with each succeeding decade. In addition, speech understanding difficulties become greater when the listening task is made more difficult. The impact of hearing loss on the elderly adversely affects both the functional health status and the psychosocial well-being of the impaired individual. It is generally thought that hearing loss can produce withdrawal, poor self-concept, depression, frustration, irritability, senility, isolation, and loneliness.

Despite the high prevalence of hearing loss among the elderly and the accepted psychosocial complications, the hearing-impaired elderly are not usually referred for audiologic intervention. Frequently, they are not considered candidates for amplification until they reach advanced old age. The reasons for this are not clear. Some elderly believe that their deafness is simply another unavoidable aspect of the aging process. This feeling lessens the person's felt need to seek rehabilitation, or the ability to justify it. These beliefs, combined with an inadequate knowledge and low expectations of rehabilitative measures, appear to discourage these individuals from seeking assistance. Even those who do seek assistance often fail to use their hearing aids to the fullest. In fact, some stop using their amplification systems soon after purchase.

The special problems of the hearing-impaired elderly require that the audiologist educate physicians and lay persons about the benefits of hearing aids. It is also important that audiologists recognize the special needs of this population. For example, during the assessment phase, one must determine whether there are any limitations in upper body movement or if arthritis exists. These conditions can interfere with an individual's ability to reach, grasp, or manipulate a hearing aid. Such information is most helpful in deciding on the type of hearing aid to be recommended. For example, a small ITC hearing aid with micro controls would be inappropriate for an individual who has arthritis affecting the hands and arms. Another important consideration in the assessment phase is the visual acuity of the patient. Like hearing, vision declines with increasing age. Since visual acuity is important for receiving auditory-visual information, it is prudent for the audiologist to assess the visual abilities of an elderly patient. This can be done simply by posing questions to the hearing-impaired person about visual status. Examples of such questions might include:

1. Do you have problems with your vision? If so, what kind?
2. Do you wear eyeglasses? Do they help you to see?

3. Are you able to see my mouth clearly?

Some audiologists actually test for far-visual acuity using the well-known Snellen eye chart.

A check for mental status is also appropriate for the elderly population. Many elderly individuals exhibit declines in cognitive function which would reduce the likelihood of successful use of a hearing aid. There are formal tests available to assess mental status. In lieu of these, however, the audiologist can simply pose questions that will offer information about the patient's cognitive functioning (i.e., memory, general knowledge, orientation). If there are problems with mental status, the audiologist will need to work closely with a "significant other" to assure appropriate use and care of the hearing aid. Other factors that need to be considered before amplification is recommended to an elderly person include motivation, family support, financial resources, and life style. Special attention is also important for the elderly during the hearing aid orientation program. Greater care is required to explain the various components of a hearing aid. Furthermore, the audiologist should schedule elderly patients for periodic follow-up visits to monitor the patients' progress and to review questions and concerns that they may have about their amplification device. When considering amplification for this group, it is important to recognize that they could benefit from many of the assistive listening devices described earlier in this chapter. Many of the problems exhibited by this group center around using the telephone, watching television, and understanding speech in group situations, such as church or public auditoriums.

To summarize, the hearing-impaired elderly have unique problems and concerns that require the special consideration of the audiologist throughout the rehabilitation process. If these needs and concerns are attended to by the audiologist, there is a far greater probability that successful use of a hearing aid will be achieved.

SUMMARY

In this chapter, we have reviewed and discussed the more pertinent issues concerned with amplification and rehabilitation of hearing-impaired children and adults. It was noted that the hearing aid is the most important rehabilitative tool we have available to us for the management of the hearing impaired. Numerous types of amplification systems, including personal hearing aids, assistive listening devices, and classroom systems, are available for the habilitation/rehabilitation of hearing-impaired individuals. Further, we have detailed in this chapter some of the varied rehabilitative approaches that have been employed for hearing-impaired children and adults.

Suggested Readings

Alpiner JG: Evaluation of adult communication function. In Alpiner JG, McCarthy PA (eds): *Rehabilitative Audiology: Children and Adults*. Baltimore, Williams & Wilkins, 1987.

Bloom L, Lahey M: *Language Development and Language Disorders*. New York, John Wiley & Sons, 1978.

Byrne D: Theoretical prescriptive approaches to selecting the gain and frequency response of a hearing aid. *Monographs in Contemporary Audiology* 4:1–40, 1983.

Fitzgerald MT, Bess FH: Parent/infant training for hearing-impaired children. *Monographs in Contemporary Audiology* 3:1–24, 1982.

Geers AE, Moog JS: Predicting spoken language acquisition of profoundly hearing impaired children. *J Speech Hear Disord* 52:84–94, 1987.

Hawkins D, Yacullo W: The signal-to-noise ratio advantage of binaural hearing aids and directional microphones under different levels of reverberation. *J Speech Hear Disord* 49:278–286, 1984.

High WS, Fairbanks G, Glorig A: Scale for self-assessment of hearing handicap. *J Speech Hear Disord* 17:321–327, 1964.

Hodgson WR (ed): *Hearing Aid Assessment and Use in Audiologic Habilitation*, ed 3. Baltimore, Williams & Wilkins, 1986.

Giolas TE, Owens E, Lamb SH, Schubert ED: Hearing performance inventory. *J Speech Hear Disord* 44:169–195, 1979.

Kretschmer RR, Kretschmer LW: Communication/language assessment of the hearing-impaired child. In Bess FH (ed), *Hearing Impairment in Children*. Parkton, MD, York Press, 1988.

Ling D: *Speech and the Hearing-Impaired Child: Theory and Practice*. Washington, DC, Alexander Graham Bell Association for the Deaf, 1976.

McCarthy P, Culpepper NB: The adult remediation process. In Alpiner JG, McCarthy PA (eds): *Rehabilitative Audiology: Children and Adults*. Baltimore, Williams & Wilkins, 1987.

Moeller MP, Brunt MA: Management of preschool hearing-impaired children: a cognitive-linguistic approach. In Bess FH (ed): *Hearing Impairment in Children*. Parkton, MD, York Press, 1988.

Moeller MP, Osberger MJ, Morford JA: Speech-language assessment and intervention with preschool hearing impaired children. In Alpiner JG, McCarthy PA (eds): *Rehabilitative Audiology: Children and Adults*. Baltimore, Williams & Wilkins, 1987.

Mueller HG, Grimes A: Amplification systems for the hearing impaired. In Alpiner JF, McCarthy PA (eds): *Rehabilitative Audiology: Children and Adults*. Baltimore, Williams & Wilkins, 1987.

Norlin PF, Van Tassell DJ: Linguistic skills of hearing-impaired children. *Monographs in Contemporary Audiology* 2:1–32, 1980.

Northern JL, Downs MP: *Hearing in Children*, ed 3. Baltimore, Williams & Wilkins, 1984.

Schwartz DM, Bess FH: Amplification techniques for hearing-impaired children. In Bluestone CD, Stool S (eds): *Pediatric Otolaryngology* ed 2. Philadelphia, WB Saunders, in press.

Skinner MW: *Hearing Aid Evaluation*. Englewood Cliffs, NJ, Prentice-Hall, 1988.

Studebaker GA, Bess FH (eds): *The Vanderbilt Hearing Aid Report*. Upper Darby, PA, Monographs in Contemporary Audiology, 1982.

CHAPTER EIGHT

Education for the Hearing Impaired

In previous chapters, reference has been made to the importance of the auditory system for acquiring information about the world. It was noted that significant hearing loss can result in serious developmental complications, such as delays in development of language, speech production and understanding, and cognition. It was also mentioned that, in the absence of hearing, the symbol system we traditionally use for developing and verbally expressing thoughts and ideas is not automatically perceived and learned. Given this background, it should come as no surprise to learn that hearing-impaired children often exhibit significant lags in educational achievement.

Education is a process of imparting to individuals information that will better prepare them for life and enable them to use their native abilities in a meaningful and constructive manner in society. When one considers the method by which information is imparted, it becomes apparent that auditory input from teacher to pupil and from pupil to pupil is critical to acquiring an education in the typical manner. Vision also plays a vital role but is secondary to hearing. One need only watch a television program without the sound to gain some realization of what hearing-impaired children experience in the classroom. Communication through hearing, so natural and automatic that it is taken for granted by most people, is reduced dramatically between a teacher and a hearing-impaired child. Many students enrolled in an introductory audiology class are likely to be faced with the responsibility of working with a hearing-impaired child later in their careers. This chapter, as a result, focuses on educational programming and the educational difficulties experienced by hearing-impaired children.

OBJECTIVES

Following completion of this chapter the reader should be able to:

- List and describe the legislative provisions for hearing-impaired children.
- Describe the different educational programs and settings available for hearing-impaired children.
- Describe the educational achievements exhibited by today's hearing-impaired children.

- Understand the impact of varying degrees of hearing loss on educational performance.
- Develop an appreciation for the role of audiology in the educational setting.

LEGISLATIVE PROVISIONS FOR HANDICAPPED CHILDREN

In 1975, Part B of the Education of the Handicapped Act (EHA) (known as the Education for All Handicapped Children Act—Public Law 94–142) was passed by Congress and signed into law. Public Law (PL) 94–142 focused on the rights and protection of handicapped children and their parents. Briefly, the law had four major functions. First, it guaranteed the availability of a special-education program to all handicapped children and youth who require it. This was true without regard for factors, such as geographic residence, that contributed to many inequities of opportunity in the past. Second, the law assured fair and appropriate decision making in providing special education to handicapped children and youth. Third, PL 94–142 established, at every level of government, clear management, auditing requirements, and procedures for special education. Fourth, the law assisted the special-education efforts of state and local governments through the use of federal funds. Importantly, the law does not mandate special education for every handicapped child, but only for those who by reason of one or more disabilities require it. Many children are able to enroll in regular classes without program modification and should do so. The law further implies that special education is "special" and includes only instruction aimed at meeting the unique needs of a handicapped child. The law also makes clear that handicapped children may require related services that might not be available from the school system itself. These services would be provided through contractual relations with other agencies, either public or private, and with outside specialists. The act demonstrates a clear and logical progression: the child is handicapped and special education and/or related services are needed by the child; special education is the specially designed instruction program to meet the child's unique needs; and related services are those additional services necessary to enable the child to benefit from special-education instruction.

In 1986, amendments were proposed which authorized the extension of the EHA to infants and toddlers, 0–2 years of age. Known as Part H of the EHA, this newly created legislation was designed to assist states in the development and implementation of comprehensive, coordinated, interdisciplinary programs of early intervention services for handicapped infants, toddlers, and their families. Children experiencing developmental delays in language and speech development are among those covered by Part H of the EHA. Early intervention services are defined as "developmental services which include . . . speech pathology and audiology . . . and are provided by qualified personnel, including speech and language pathologists and audiologists" (1). Other services targeted by the bill include early identification, screening, and assessment services; psychological services; medical services for diagnostic or evaluation purposes only; and any other services deemed appropriate for helping infants and toddlers benefit from early intervention. In addition, the bill strengthens portions of the original act by developing better incentives for states to serve the 3- to 5-year old population. Finally, not only does the bill help to expand the services to young infants and toddlers but it also helps to ensure that states use appropriately trained personnel.

In consideration of this bill, now known as Public Law 99–457, Congress recognized a need to:

"1. enhance the development of handicapped infants and toddlers and to minimize their potential for developmental delay;

2. reduce the educational costs to our society, including our Nation's schools, by minimizing the need for special education and related services after handicapped infants and toddlers reach school age;

3. minimize the likelihood of institutionalization of handicapped individuals and maximize the potential for their independent living in society; and

4. enhance the capacity of families to meet the special needs of their infants and toddlers with handicaps"[1].

COMMUNICATION MODES USED IN EDUCATIONAL INSTRUCTION

In Chapter 7, we discussed briefly the different modes of communication used for educational instruction: auditory-oral and total communication. It is not our intent here to suggest that one mode of communication is better than another. Unquestionably, the two most common approaches used in education are the auditory-oral and total communication methods. Recall that the auditory-oral method, sometimes referred to as the oral-aural approach, places emphasis on using the child's existing residual hearing to develop oral communication. Some of the advocates of this method use early amplification with no emphasis on vision for receiving information. Others emphasize vision over hearing or stress the combined use of audition and vision equally. Whatever modification is used, this approach does not allow for the use of signs or finger spelling. The only means of expression allowed is speech.

The other popular approach to educational instruction is the method known as total communication. Total communication combines the auditory-oral method with signs and finger spelling. That is, the emphasis is on receiving the information by all possible means, including amplification, vision, signs, and finger spelling. Similarly, expression can occur by speech or through signs and/ or finger spelling. Like advocates of the auditory-oral approach, proponents of total communication believe that the method should be introduced in early infancy, if possible, and parents should be intensively involved. The difference, of course, is that with total communication, the parents assist the child in the development of language using all means available.

The auditory-oral method was easily the most widely used method of instruction until the mid-1970s. Since that time, however, total communication has become the more popular method and is used in about 70% of the educational programs in the United States, regardless of grade level. This approach gained widespread acceptance following research that showed that deaf children, exposed to manual communication by deaf parents, exhibited better educational performance than deaf children of hearing parents. At the same time, the two groups of children showed essentially no differences in their speech.

At this point, a brief discussion of manual communication is warranted, since it is an important component of the total approach. Manual communication is the expression of words and phrases through the movement of the hands and fingers. A common way in which to accomplish this is through finger spelling. Finger spelling simply involves spelling a word letter by letter, representing each letter by a specific sign that corresponds to a letter in the English alphabet. The hand is held at about chest level, and different finger configurations are then formed. The presentation rate is somewhat similar to that of speech. The American manual alphabet used in the United States is shown in Figure 8.1. Note that there are 26 handshapes representing the different letters in the English alphabet.

The second means by which a word or idea can be presented manually is through the use of sign. There are four basic features common to all signs. These

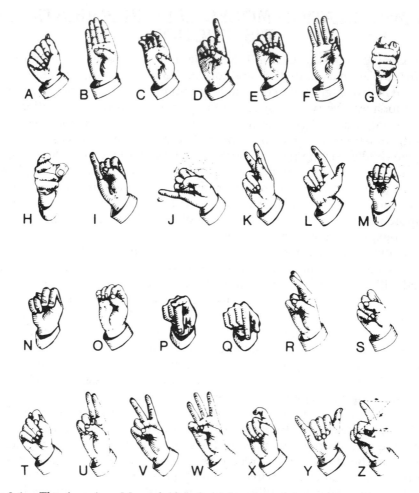

Figure 8.1. The American Manual Alphabet (shown as signs appear to person reading them). (From Schleper D: *Communicating with Deaf People: An Introduction*. Washington, DC, National Information Center on Deafness, Gallaudet University, 1987.)

include general position, configuration, orientation (direction of the palms), and movement of the hands. These four features are combined in various ways to formulate signs of different meanings. Examples of signs are shown in Figure 8.2. Although the different signs in this figure all use the same handshape, the movement, position, and palm orientation alter the meaning. The manual communicator has the flexibility to use finger spelling only, sign only, or a combination of the two. Finger spelling is considered the more formal language, since it is more like English than sign. The sign language used in the United States is generally referred to as American Sign Language (ASL), to differentiate it from some of the more recent modifications devised to make signs conform more closely to the syntax of the English language. Varying forms of sign language developed to bring ASL in closer relation to English include Manual English, Signed English, Visual English, and Seeing Essential English (SEE). Each is based on ASL but employs the word order of English. Signed English consists of both signs and finger spelling. Manual English and SEE add morphemes such as prefixes and suffixes that are not included in the basic signs. Examples include the morphemes -*ed*, as in "talk*ed*," and -*ly*, as in "friend*ly*." Visual English also uses ASL vocabulary, supplemented by a vocabulary of morphemes. Those who desire a more detailed coverage of manual communication are referred to the sources listed in the Suggested Readings at the end of this chapter.

There are other, less common approaches used in instruction. One technique

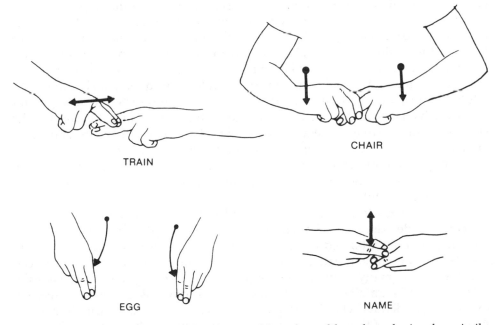

TRAIN

CHAIR

EGG

NAME

Figure 8.2. Examples of a group of signs. Note that, although each sign has similar handshapes, there are differences in movement, placement, and orientation of the hands. (From Schleper D: *Communicating with Deaf People: An Introduction.* Washington, DC, National Information Center on Deafness, Gallaudet University, 1987.)

for instruction is the Rochester Method, established at the Rochester School for the Deaf many years ago. This technique attempted to overcome the syntactic deficiencies of sign language by using the manual alphabet, or finger spelling, simultaneously with speech. Another approach is cued speech. Cued speech is a system that incorporates eight hand configurations and four hand positions near the lips to serve as aids to hearing and speech reading. The basic premise is that the hand cues can supplement speechreading and audition by signalling differences between sounds. For example, the words *bee* and *me* look alike to the speech reader. A hand cue made simultaneously at the lips signals the difference between the two "look-alike" words.

TYPES OF EDUCATIONAL SETTINGS

What are the different types of settings used to educate hearing-impaired children? There are numerous types of programs, both public and private, designed to serve hearing-impaired children of all ages. One of the most well recognized types of educational program is the residential school. Residential programs maintain facilities for room and board as well as instruction and recreation. Most residential schools are operated by state governments. There are, however, some well-known private residential programs located throughout the United States. Today, many children commute on a daily basis to residential facilities, especially if the school is located in a metropolitan area. Also found in large metropolitan areas are private and public day schools for the hearing impaired. In these schools, the hearing-impaired children commute on a daily basis like normal-hearing children. Day classes represent another type of instructional format for hearing-impaired children. Here, classes for the hearing impaired are conducted in public schools where most of the children have normal hearing. Instruction may take place entirely in classrooms containing only hearing-impaired students, or the children may be "mainstreamed." Mainstreaming refers to the integration of hearing-impaired children into regular classrooms on a full-time or part-time basis. Special classes (resource rooms) are arranged for areas in which the child needs individualized tutorial assistance, but most of the student's time is spent in regular classrooms. Finally, there are itinerant programs, in which a hearing-impaired child attends regular classrooms full time but receives support services from an itinerant teacher. Typically, the itinerant teacher moves from one school to another throughout the week, offering support services to those children with special needs.

It is of interest to consider how these placement alternatives have changed over the past decade. Figure 8.3 contrasts the different types of programs hearing-impaired children attended in 1974 with the educational programs attended in 1984. Several enrollment patterns are observed in this figure. First, it can be seen that there were many more hearing-impaired children in public day classes in 1984 than in 1974. Paralleling the increase in public day classes was a decrease in the public residential schools and public day schools for the hearing impaired. Also noteworthy is the decrease in all types of private schools throughout the United States. Between 1974 and 1984, there was a trend toward an increase in the role of the public schools in educating the hearing impaired, mostly through day-school programs (public day classes). This trend is no doubt due to the

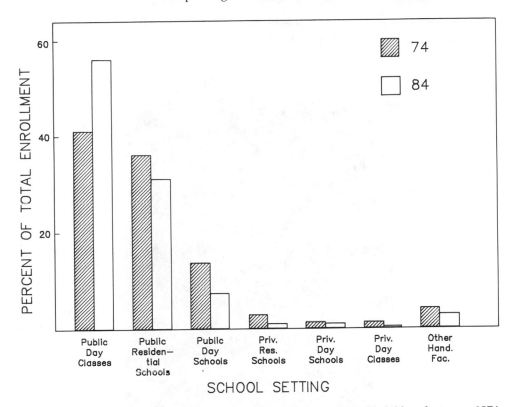

Figure 8.3. Differences in school enrollment of hearing-impaired children between 1974 and 1984. (Adapted from Moores DF: *Educating the Deaf—Psychology, Principles and Practices,* ed. 3. Boston, Houghton Mifflin, 1987.)

mandate of Public Law 94–142 in 1975 and will continue to increase with the recent passage of Public Law 99–457.

There are a number of postsecondary educational opportunities available for the deaf and hard-of-hearing population in the United States. Foremost is Gallaudet University, which was for many years the only higher educational program in the world developed specifically for the hearing impaired. The establishment of the university was spearheaded by the efforts of Edward Minor Gallaudet and Amos Kendall, two resourceful professionals who were committed to serving the hearing-impaired population. The university was named after Edward Gallaudet's father, Thomas Gallaudet, a pioneer in deaf education. (See Vignette 8.1 for a discussion of pioneers in deaf education.) Today, Gallaudet serves as a major source of leadership to the hearing-impaired population in the United States. In addition to offering liberal arts and graduate education for the hearing impaired, Gallaudet also trains professionals such as school administrators, audiologists, speech-language pathologists, teachers, and researchers to serve the hearing-impaired population. There is no comparable postsecondary program for the hearing-impaired population in the United States.

Technical schools for the hearing impaired also exist in this country. Perhaps the best known is the National Technical Institute for the Deaf (NTID), a technical school of higher education that serves deaf students in association with the

Vignette 8.1.   Pioneers in Deaf Education

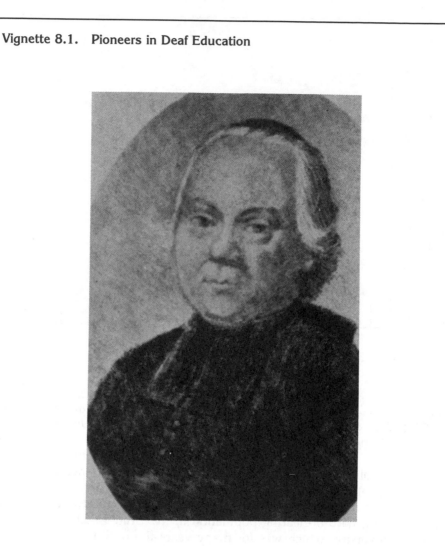

Charles Michael de l'Pée

One of the most prominent names in the history of deaf education, worldwide, is that of Abbé de l'Pée, the individual credited with making education of the hearing-impaired a matter of public concern. He was also interested in making education available to the indigent population. Charles Michael de l'Pée was born in Versailles, France, in 1712. He was well educated and pursued the priesthood as his chosen profession. His interest in deafness stemmed from his knowledge of twin sisters who were severe-to-profoundly hearing impaired. Because of his concern for these sisters, he agreed to provide them with instruction, and soon his success gained him widespread recognition. From this time on he devoted his life to working with the hearing impaired. He established a school, and educators from all over the world came to study his technique. Also de l'Pée helped develop and expand the sign language for the hearing impaired and served as an advocate for manual communication.

Vignette 8.1   (Continued)

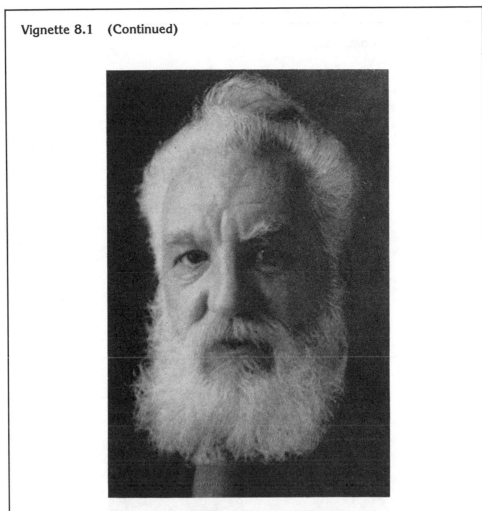

Alexander Graham Bell

Alexander Graham Bell is recognized as one of the great teachers of the deaf in the United States. He was born March 3, 1847, in Edinburgh, Scotland. At 24 years of age, he came to the United States to visit a school for deaf children. He was most impressed with how hearing-impaired children utilized lipreading and speech. This initial experience motivated Bell to become more involved with the hearing impaired. Bell spearheaded the development of the auditory-oral method for teaching the deaf in the United States. In 1872, he opened a training school for teachers of the deaf in Boston, Massachusetts. His plan to develop an auditory-oral training school was met with great opposition by advocates of the manual approach. His desire to develop a mechanical means of making speech visible to the hearing impaired led Bell to experiment with the electrical transmission of sound. He hoped to develop a means of amplification for the hearing impaired. These experiments resulted in the development of the telephone. Bell later married Mabel Hubbard, a deaf woman who helped start the auditory-oral approach in the United States. Throughout his later years, Bell maintained his interest in the education of the hearing impaired and served as an advocate for the hearing-impaired population.

Vignette 8.1   (Continued)

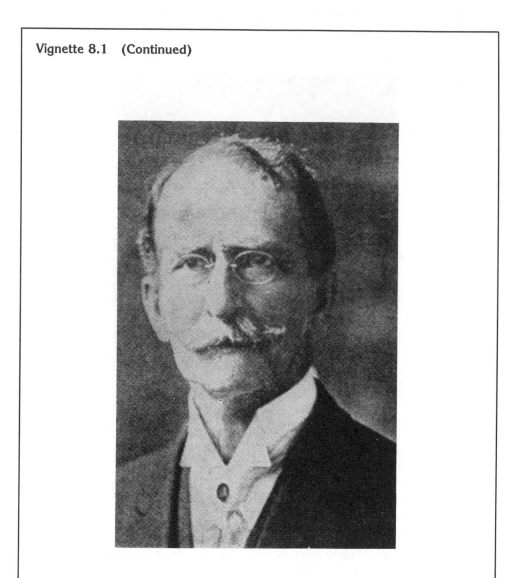

Edward Minor Gallaudet

Edward Minor Gallaudet was the son of Thomas Hopkins Gallaudet, a pioneering teacher of the hearing impaired in the United States and the man for whom Gallaudet University in Washington, D.C., was named. Edward Minor Gallaudet studied under his father and served as the first president of Kendall School, a private school for the hearing impaired. The school was later renamed Gallaudet College in honor of Thomas Hopkins Gallaudet. Kendall School became the preparatory department at this college. Edward Minor Gallaudet studied both oral and manual techniques; he supported the combined method but was convinced that manual communication was the most appropriate and natural approach for the educational instruction of hearing-impaired children.

Rochester Institute of Technology in Rochester, New York. The educational programs can lead to certificate programs, associate degrees, or bachelor's degrees. NTID is also involved in carrying out research concerned with the deaf and hard-of-hearing populations.

Finally, it is important to note that there are a number of state universities and community colleges throughout the United States that have federally funded programs providing vocational or liberal arts training to the hearing impaired. In fact, some of these programs serve as feeder programs for NTID and Gallaudet University.

EDUCATIONAL ACHIEVEMENT OF HEARING-IMPAIRED CHILDREN

One only needs to contrast the manner in which a normal-hearing child develops oral speech and language with the situation of the hearing-impaired child to appreciate the learning difficulties that children with auditory deficits experience. The normal-hearing child comes to kindergarten or first grade with a wide array of auditory experiences and a well-developed language symbol system. The hearing-impaired child, on the other hand, has had limited auditory experiences and was most likely not even identified as suffering from hearing loss until 3 years of age. Therefore, the hearing-impaired child will have been wearing hearing aids for only 1 or 2 years. The child with a significant hearing impairment will have had far fewer learning-readiness experiences prior to entering first grade. Thus, we find that children with hearing loss lag behind normal-hearing children in educational achievement.

Indeed, both education and communication are reflected in the incomes earned by the deaf population. Those with the most education generally earn the highest incomes. Those using only manual communication or gestures report the lowest median earnings. Of those in the upper half of the income range, about 90% use speech to communicate at work, with about half using speech combined with one or more other modes of communication and half using speech exclusively.

Although we find that unemployment rates among the deaf are higher on the average than in the hearing population, underemployment is a much more serious problem. For example, less than 10% are employed in professional, technical, or managerial positions, and less than 1% in sales. Almost 75% are engaged in clerical, craft, or machine operator positions—the latter being the single largest occupation. Some of the reasons for underemployment will become apparent as we review the educational difficulties experienced by children with varying degrees of hearing loss. The case illustrations of four different school-age hearing-impaired children presented in Vignettes 8.2, 8.3, 8.4, and 8.5 will also provide some insight into the problem.

Children with Severe-to-Profound Hearing Losses

In general terms, there appears to be an association between the severity of hearing loss and the degree of educational retardation. The milder the hearing loss, however, the more difficult it is to predict the educational potential of the child. Since the 1920s, it has been acknowledged that deafness causes an

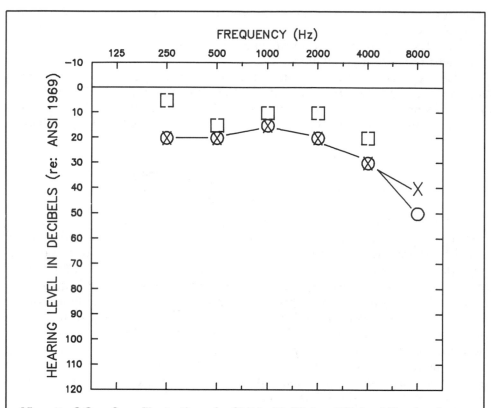

Vignette 8.2.   Case Illustration of a Child with Bilateral Minimal Hearing Loss

This child is a 6-year-old male with a long history of middle ear disease with effusion. He has had persistent otitis media for several years and a history of myringotomy with insertion tubes beginning at the age of 6 months. The child has had seven or eight sets of tubes during the first 6 years of life. He was hospitalized a total of 22 times for difficult-to-resolve otitis media and he received a mastoidectomy and tympanoplasty on the right side.

It is noted from the audiogram that the child has a very mild hearing impairment bilaterally through the speech frequency range and a somewhat precipitous drop in the high frequencies in the right ear. The child experienced considerable difficulty understanding speech in a background of noise. That is, when tested in a sound field situation in the presence of background noise (+6 S:N), the child was only able to understand 76% of the speech material.

He is currently enrolled in kindergarten, where he is having considerable difficulty. There is serious question as to whether he will progress to the first grade. He is reportedly immature and hyperactive. Language skills, especially vocabulary, are delayed by 1–2 years.

Based on these results, a number of recommendations were made: (*a*) that he continue with otologic management for middle ear disease with effusion; (*b*) that he receive support in the form of an FM system for use in the academic setting (this system was recommended to improve the S:N ratio in the noisy classroom environment); (*c*) that the Board of Education be notified of the child's circumstance so that the audiologic and academic needs of the child can be monitored; and (*d*) that the child be seen by the audiologist on a 6-month basis to monitor progress.

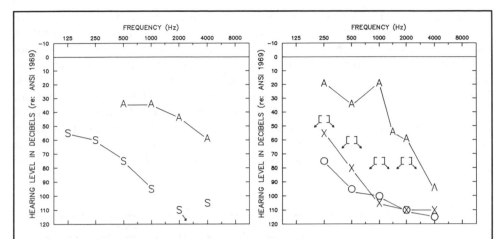

Vignette 8.3. Case Illustration of a Child with Bilateral Moderately Severe to Profound Sensorineural Hearing Loss

This 10-year-old male was identified at the age of 17 months as having a moderately severe to profound sensorineural hearing loss bilaterally. Binaural amplification was introduced within a month, and an audiogram obtained after 2 months of amplification is shown in the accompanying figure (*left panel*). Thresholds obtained in a sound field (*S-S*) reveal a severe-to-profound hearing loss. When the child wears a hearing aid, the sound field thresholds (*A-A*) are seen to improve markedly when compared to unaided thresholds. A recent pure-tone audiogram is shown in the *right panel*. Data for aided thresholds are also presented.

He was enrolled in an auditory-oral parent-infant training program as soon as amplification was introduced. His parents were taught speech, language, and auditory stimulation techniques and were excellent in carrying out auditory training at home. The child progressed rapidly and was making single-word approximations accompanied by jargon at 1 year post-amplification.

At 3 years of age, he was enrolled in a half-day oral-acoustic nursery for hearing-impaired children. He wore an FM-wireless system during school hours. By 5 years of age, he was using simple sentences to communicate (orally), and he was mainstreamed into a private prekindergarten classroom with supportive services from the local school. The support services consisted of individual speech and language therapy as well as assistance in the curricular areas of reading, math, science, and social studies.

The subject continues to be mainstreamed in a private school, with supportive speech and language therapy. He is presently in the third grade and functioning at grade level in reading comprehension and math. He is functioning below age level in the areas of vocabulary development and language associated with logical thinking skills (i.e., sequencing events, predicting outcomes, verbal analogies, and multiple meanings).

Intelligibility of speech production is good, with approximately 90% of his speech understood by peers, teachers, and family members. The child orally presents essays and other assignments on a par with other children in his class.

He probably will require speech/langage therapy throughout his school years, as well as special assistance with academic subjcts. However, this is a case where appropriate early identification combined with proper educational management and parental determination has led to a life in the mainstream.

educational lag of 4–5 years. This lowered achievement is thought to result from the difficulty children experience in acquiring language and communication skills. Delayed speech and language in the important preschool years cannot help but be reflected when a child learns to read, since reading achievement is an important indicator of linguistic competence. Reading constitutes a basic learning tool that directly influences the mastery of all other academic content. For years, educators of deaf children have been concerned with the apparent "plateau effect" that begins at about 9–10 years of age and persists through the teens. This effect is reflected in very minimal gains in reading level over several years of instruction. For example, the average gain in reading between 10 and 16

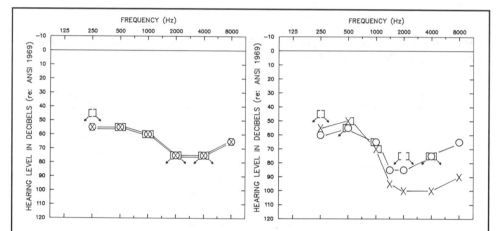

Vignette 8.4.   Case Illustration of a Child with Bilateral Moderate-to-Severe Sensorineural Hearing Loss

This 11-year-old female was identified as having a moderate-to-severe sensorineural hearing loss bilaterally at age 5 years and was referred to a hearing clinic. The etiology of the hearing loss is unknown. Her audiogram at age 5 is shown in the accompanying figure (*left panel*). The most recent audiogram indicated a moderate-to-severe sensorineural hearing loss in the right ear and a moderate-to-profound sensorineural hearing loss in the left ear (*right panel*).

The child was enrolled in a self-contained kindergarten classroom in a local school system and, in addition, in a parent-infant training program. Her communicative skills were fair, and she responded well to amplification. Her speech was judged to be partially intelligible, and her language skills were similar to those of a 3- to 4-year-old. She has continued in a self-contained classroom with additional individual speech/language therapy. She is presently in a second-grade self-contained classroom. Her reading skills are at age level, and she is functioning at grade level in math and social sciences. When compared to normal-hearing children, expressive language skills are at the 7-year-old level.

Mainstreaming has been considered but has not been implemented due to concerns regarding her ability to work independently. In addition, mainstreaming has been prevented due to lack of qualified personnel to provide the necessary support services. It is probable that she will be mainstreamed, at least partially, when she is older and more able to work independently.

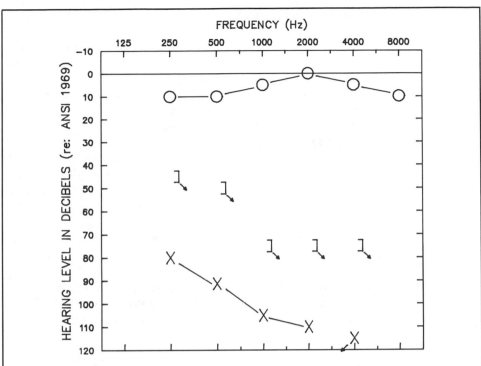

Vignette 8.5. Case Illustration of a Child with Unilateral Severe-to-Profound Sensorineural Hearing Loss

This child is a 6-year-old male with a severe-to-profound sensorineural hearing loss in the left ear and normal hearing in the right ear. Pertinent medical history includes maternal diabetes and syphilis, meningitis at 1 year of age, and head trauma at 5 years of age. He is currently attending first grade and receives preferential seating (child seated to the right side of the teacher so that the good ear is fully exposed to the teacher). The teacher had indicated that he would be retained in the first grade for the next year. She reported that he is a "slow learner," although he is more capable than he demonstrates. He also attends a reading resource class and receives articulation therapy.

Prior to a 2-week trial with an FM system, the teacher rated his ability to understand and/or follow directions as "fair" in small group situations and as "very poor" in large group situations. The teacher also rated his ability to concentrate on tasks as "poor."

Use of an FM wireless system reportedly resulted in a marked improvement in his performance. His ability to understand and/or follow directions in small and large group situations as well as his ability to concentrate on tasks while using the FM wireless system was now rated by the teacher as "good." In addition the teacher felt that peer acceptance of the FM wireless system was excellent. According to the teacher, the FM wireless system was especially useful in classroom learning situations.

Both the teachers and the parents were counseled about the dangers that unilaterally hearing-impaired children can encounter relative to such routine activities as crossing busy streets and bike riding in heavy traffic. In addition, the teachers and the parents were counseled about the need for practicing good hearing health care. Monitoring the child for possible conductive hearing loss resulting from effusion in either ear and progressive sensorineural hearing loss was emphasized. Furthermore, the practice of using ear protection in any type of high-noise environment was recommended as a conservation measure.

years of age among deaf students is less than a year. One can expect profoundly hearing-impaired children to be retarded 7–8 years in reading vocabulary by the age of 18 years. There are, however, many exceptions.

There have been a number of national surveys on the hearing-impaired population. In a 1974 census of deaf individuals who could not hear and understand speech and who had lost that ability by 19 years of age (or never had it), it was found that 52% had not completed high school and 25–33% had not completed the ninth grade. Although such data should be interpreted with caution, since it reports years completed and not achievement level, it does offer insight into some of the educational difficulties experienced by the deaf population. In another survey, conducted by the Office of Demographic Studies at Gallaudet University, more than 19,000 hearing-impaired children and youth were evaluated for educational achievement using appropriate test measures for this population. The data are more representative of the severely and profoundly impaired, since two-thirds were in educational programs designed exclusively for hearing-impaired children. Some of the results from selected subtests of the reading achievement test for 9-year-olds and 13-year-olds are presented in Figure 8.4. The grade expectancy for normal children is also provided for comparison.

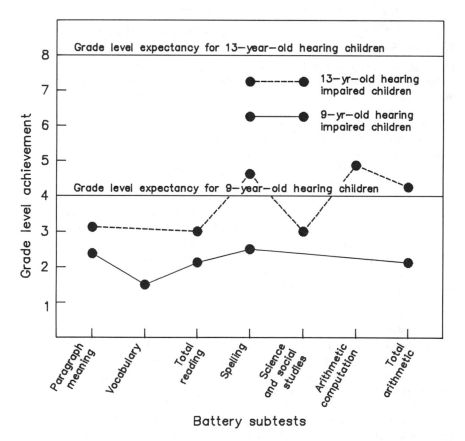

Figure 8.4.   Average grade level achievement attained by two groups of hearing-impaired children on subtests of the Stanford Achievement Test.

The data, summarized in Figure 8.4, clearly illustrate the educational lag that is common to deaf and partially hearing children enrolled in our special programs. While the younger children at 9 years are retarded about 2 years in grade level, the children at 13 years have fallen even farther behind and are retarded more than 4 years. For the 13-year-old hearing-impaired children, the highest level of performance occurs on the spelling and arithmetic computation subtests. Competency in spelling does not require the language proficiency needed for reading comprehension and can be acquired by the visual mode. Similarly, arithmetic computation skills are not highly dependent on language. However, the mean reported for the arithmetic concepts subtest, although not included here, is much lower, reflecting the influence of verbal comprehension. The total arithmetic mean grade level shown in Figure 8.4 is reduced by more than half a grade because of this effect.

Children with Mild-to-Moderate Hearing Losses

Thus far, our discussion has focused on the impact of severe-to-profound hearing losses on education. What about children suffering from the milder forms of hearing loss, sometimes referred to as the hard-of-hearing or the partially hearing-impaired population? Once again, we find that even those with milder hearing losses can experience difficulty in school. In 1968, researchers examined the educational potential of 116 hearing-impaired children using subtests of the Stanford Achievement Test. The results from this study are summarized in Table 8.1. This table shows the differences between expected performance (computed from the birthdates of the children) and actual performance for children with varying degrees of hearing loss on the subtests of word meaning, paragraph meaning, and language. Several important points are evident from this table. First, it is noted that there is a slight trend toward decreasing IQ with increasing hearing loss. Second, all groups of hearing-impaired children, even those with

Table 8.1.
Differences between Expected and Actual Performance of Children on the Stanford Achievement Test[a]

Average Hearing Threshold Level (Better Ear) in dB	No. of Children	IQ	Word Meaning[b]	Paragraph Meaning[b]	Language[b]	Subtest Average[b]
< 15	59	105.14	−1.04	−0.47	−0.78	−0.73
15–26	37	100.81	−1.40	−0.86	−1.16	−1.11
27–40	6	103.50	−3.48	−1.78	−1.95	−2.31
41–55	9	97.89	−3.84	−2.54	−2.93	−3.08
56–70	5	92.40	−2.78	−2.20	−3.52	−2.87

[a]From Quigley SP: *Some Effects of Hearing Impairment upon School Performance.* Springfield, IL, Division of Special Education Services, Department of Special Education Development and Education, 1968.
[b]Negative values repesent a deficit in measured grade level compared to normal-hearing children.

losses as mild as 15–26 dB, exhibited lags in educational performance. This is indicated by the appearance of negative numbers in the table. Third, one can see by looking at the subtest averages that the discrepancy between expected performance and actual performance increases with increasing hearing loss. The average difference between expected performance and actual performance for all groups was −1.25 grades. These data, although not universally acknowledged, demonstrate that children with slight hearing impairments are not achieving at levels consistent with their potential.

The data in Table 8.1 prompted other investigators to explore the impact of milder hearing losses on educational achievement. Foremost in this effort has been the work of Davis and coworkers published in 1981 and in 1986. Davis and coworkers conducted two comprehensive studies on the educational abilities of hearing-impaired children in the schools. In the first study, data were taken from the school files of more than 1000 children with mild to moderately severe hearing impairments. The findings of this retrospective study revealed that the children with mild-to-moderate degrees of hearing loss (three-frequency pure tone average of ≤50 dB) did not show significant educational problems. Those with average hearing losses of >50 dB, however, exhibited significant deficits in academic achievement, and these problems increased over time. In contrast, most of the hearing-impaired children, even those with mild losses, demonstrated difficulties with language.

In a follow-up investigation, a prospective study was performed on a group of 40 children with mild to moderately severe hearing losses. Rather than rely on test scores from the school files, as before, all subjects in the sample were administered the same battery of educational achievement tests. Importantly, and in contrast to the previous study, it was not possible to predict educational performance on the basis of just hearing level. That is, it was possible for a child with minimal hearing loss to exhibit as much difficulty with a given task as a child with a mild-to-moderate hearing loss, or even more difficulty. The difficulties experienced by these children could be lumped into three general areas: verbal skills, academic skills, and social development. Verbal skills appeared to be affected most, and this area was also reported to be the most closely associated with hearing loss. These researchers emphasized the heterogeneity of the hearing-impaired population and concluded that "children with any degree of hearing loss appear to be at risk for delayed development of verbal skills and reduced academic achievement"[2].

Another important finding of this study was that many of these children exhibited behavioral problems. Many were also concerned about peer acceptance. One of the children from the study related the following: "I don't have very many friends. Oh, people say, 'Hi, Kris, hi, Kris,' but only 'Hi, Kris,' never anything—you know—go out for lunch or go out on dates or anything like that. The only friends I almost have are my teachers and my counselors"[2].

Children with Unilateral Sensorineural Hearing Losses

Not only are children with mild hearing loss at risk, but it appears that children with unilateral sensorineural hearing loss also experience difficulty in the schools. The auditory, linguistic, and psychoeducational skills of a group of school-age children with unilateral sensorineural hearing loss have been examined extensively in recent years. Some of the important findings of this recent research include the following:

1. In a survey of 60 children with unilateral hearing loss, 35% were found to have failed at least one grade in the schools, and an additional 13% needed special resource assistance.
2. Children with unilateral sensorineural hearing loss exhibited greater difficulty than children with normal hearing in understanding speech in the presence of a competing background of noise.
3. Children with unilateral sensorineural hearing loss experienced significantly greater problems with localization of sound.
4. Children with severe-to-profound unilateral hearing loss exhibited lower IQs than those children with milder unilateral loss.
5. Children with unilateral sensorineural hearing loss who failed a grade in elementary school exhibited verbal IQs that were significantly lower than unilaterally hearing-impaired children who had not failed a grade.
6. Teachers rated children with unilateral losses as having greater difficulty in peer relations, less social confidence, greater likelihood of "acting out" or withdrawn behavior in the classroom, greater frustration and dependence on the teacher, and more frequent distractibility.

Historically, prior to this research, the prevailing belief had been that unilaterally hearing-impaired children do not experience any problems in the schools. It has always been assumed that one good ear is sufficient to enable a child to achieve satisfactorily in school.

Children with Mild Conductive Losses from Otitis Media

For almost 2 decades, there has been a growing awareness of the potential psychoeducational complications associated with recurrent otitis media (ROM) during the early developmental years. Although many of the research studies conducted in this area have flaws in design, the vast majority of such studies imply a linkage between a history of ROM, associated hearing loss, and some area of child development. Otitis-proneness in children has been linked to learning disabilities, academic problems, lower intelligence levels, behavior and attention problems, difficulties in understanding speech in a background of noise, and delayed language development.

How is it that the mild, fluctuating hearing loss associated with OM could possibly interfere with the development of auditory, linguistic, and psychoeducational skills? Recall from Chapter 5 that children with OM experience hearing loss averaging about 30 dB through the speech-frequency range. During the early developmental period for speech and language, the otitis-prone child could experience an inconsistent, and perhaps a somewhat distorted, auditory signal. In fact, many of the speech sounds that have low speech energy, such as /f/, /s/, /θ/, /k/, /p/, /h/, /z/, and /v/, may well be missed altogether in the presence of a mild 30-dB hearing loss. Similarly, important acoustic information, such as morphologic markers (i.e., plural -s, past tense -ed) and inflections could be especially difficult to identify.

The loss of acoustic energy explains, in part, how these children could experience trouble in the developmental years. Once the otitis-prone years have passed, can the child make up for the lost input? Unfortunately, there is some evidence to suggest that some children do not. OM can produce both delays in language and an inattention to language. Once the OM resolves or the episodes become less frequent, the child can recover basic language skills, but the habit of not attending to language may persist. Some of the more basic language components, such as syntax and semantics, may not be as seriously affected as discourse and narrative skills. The latter require some amount of attention to language.

AUDIOLOGY IN THE SCHOOLS

We have just seen that children with varying degrees of hearing loss undergo a considerable hardship in school and typically lag behind their normal-hearing peers in terms of academic achievement. The audiologist can play an important role in the management of these children in the schools. The following discussion focuses on the role of the audiologist in the educational setting.

Models for Delivering Audiologic Services to the Schools

The delivery of audiologic services within the educational environment varies considerably from one local educational agency (LEA) to the next. Educational systems offer programs ranging from comprehensive audiologic management to only minimal services. While numerous models exist for the provision of audiologic management to the schools, there are three commonly employed approaches. These models include the *parent-referral approach*, a *cooperative interagency approach*, and an *audiology program within the schools*.

Parent-Referral Model

The parent-referral model is the most traditional approach to the delivery of audiologic services in the schools. The LEA provides identification and intervention services, while the more comprehensive assessment and evaluation services are supplied by agencies or parties outside of the LEA. The success of this model is highly dependent on the parents, who become responsible for the management and follow-up of their child. Once the parents have been notified by the school that their child has been identified by the screening process as being in need of further testing, they must then make arrangements on their own for an audiologic or medical evaluation. The results of these evaluations are given directly to the parent, with feedback supplied to the LEA.

The advantages to this model are that services are provided at a minimal cost to the LEA and that the school system uses resources that already exist within the community, avoiding unnecessary duplication of services. Unfortunately, there are more disadvantages to the parent-referral model than advantages. The LEA has no control over the management of a child and must rely on the cooperation of the parent, the hearing and speech center, and the physician to supply the necessary information and recommendations. Since the LEA does not monitor referred children, many complications can arise. For example, there is no mechanism for ensuring that diagnostic reports will be sent to the school within a reasonable period of time or that they will be sent at all. In addition, the received reports may be incomplete or perhaps inappropriate in that the information provided may not assist the school or teacher in helping the child educationally. Seldom does the report supply sufficient information relative to the child's educational placement and/or management. Even if such information were available, the model provides no assurance that the child will receive appropriate follow-up. Finally, the parent-referral model is only conducive to an annual evaluation and not to continuous audiologic management.

Cooperative Interagency Model

A more desirable alternative to the provision of audiologic services in the schools is a contractual arrangement between the LEA and a community hearing and speech center. Once the child is identified, the school notifies the parents and the contract agency. Although dependent on the contracted services, the agency ordinarily provides audiologic management of the child and maintains constant feedback to an LEA designate, usually the coordinator of the program for the hearing impaired. In some instances, an audiologist coordinates the referral and management activities. The parent initiates a referral to the physician, if necessary, at the recommendation of the school. The physician, in turn, provides feedback to the parent, school, and contract agency.

The success of this model is dependent on the types of services contracted. The more knowledgeable the administrator, the more comprehensive the contract will be and the more success the model will have. The agreement works best when an audiologist from the agency is solely responsible for coordinating the audiologic services. The contact person at the LEA and the teachers must have one person to whom they can refer questions or problems.

The model offers several advantages and eliminates some of the disadvantages associated with the parent-referral model. It is particularly useful for educational systems with small numbers of hearing- impaired children (such as schools located in rural areas). Duplication of services is avoided, and, as with the parent-referral model, the LEA does not need to be concerned with the high cost of equipment and facilities. At a time when funding is a primary concern in education, this must be considered a distinct advantage. There are also several limitations inherent in this model. Unless responsibilities and lines of authority are clearly defined and monitored on a continuing basis, communication breakdown can occur. Since the LEA is paying for the audiologic services, there is a tendency for the educational administration to dictate the type and extent of services to be provided. Open lines of communication, willingness to cooperate with the LEA staff, and general agreement on services to be delivered are essential. Another potential difficulty is the LEA's loss of control over expenditures, although this problem can be eliminated by carefully defining in the contract how funds will be expended.

School Audiology Model

The final model involves the development of a comprehensive audiologic program within the LEA. In this model, services are provided by a coordinating audiologist and associated staff. This model provides the LEA with complete centralized control of audiologic services. Identification, assessment, and management are all under the jurisdiction of the coordinating school audiologist. The advantage to such a model is that the audiologist is located where the children are—in the schools. Individualized educational programs (IEPs) for the hearing-impaired students can be developed and implemented in the schools. Effective input to these plans would be difficult for professionals outside the system. Other advantages of this model include immediate access to diagnostic information, development of evaluation data tailored to the educational setting, greater control over follow-up, good communication between the LEA staff and the school audiologist, and better potential for ongoing in-service education. The limitations of the model are the high costs of equipping a complete audiologic facility and employing the needed personnel and the problems that arise from duplicating services that are already available within the community. Now that we have reviewed three of the models used for delivering services to the schools, let us briefly examine some of the responsibilities of the school audiologist.

Responsibilities of Audiologists in the Schools

The duties of the audiologist in the school setting are numerous and require highly specialized skills and knowledge. These responsibilities include identification, assessment, audiologic management, educational admission and placement, and in-service training.

Identification

Ideally, the educational audiologist should have primary responsibility for the identification of preschool and school-age children with hearing loss or middle ear disease. Even if identification services are not offered directly by the school program, the educational audiologist should coordinate the screening program. Techniques for setting up screening programs have been discussed in Chapter 6.

Assessment

A major responsibility of the educational audiologist is to assess the communicative efficiency of hearing-impaired children in the schools. The assessment battery should include traditional measurements of auditory function (pure-tone audiometry, speech audiometry, and immittance measures) as well as the evaluation of auditory processing and communicative skills. Assessment protocols have been addressed elsewhere in this book.

Audiologic Management

The school audiologist plays an important role in the audiologic management of the hearing-impaired child. The associated responsibilities might include selection and evaluation of amplification and assistive listening devices, maintenance of amplification devices, monitoring classroom noise, coordination of habilitation/rehabilitation activities, and parent counseling.

Educational Admission and Placement

The audiologist should be an active member of the staff that reviews a child's school status for the purpose of deciding placement or admission. The audiologist's input should be evident in the individual education program (IEP) as it relates to amplification needs, the amount and type of language and speech intervention required, the acoustic classroom environment, parent and child counseling, and support systems for the classroom teacher. Unfortunately, the audiologist is generally not included in the IEP unless specifically requested by the parent or teacher.

In-Service Education

An important responsibility of the audiologist in the schools is the development of in-service education programs for school personnel who come in frequent contact with hearing-impaired children. In addition to providing in-service training to speech-language pathologists and teachers of the hearing impaired, more generalized in-service programs should be developed for regular teachers, psychologists, administrators, and support personnel. Teachers of the hearing impaired whose previous experience was confined to the self-contained classroom are now being asked to service hearing-impaired children either in a resource room or as an itinerant teacher. In addition, support personnel who previously only encountered children with mild-to-moderate hearing loss are now faced with the task of mainstreaming severely-to-profoundly hearing-impaired children. Many educators find themselves needing to upgrade and broaden their skills in order to meet the demands of hearing-impaired children and comply with the provisions of Public Laws 94–142 and 99–457.

SUMMARY

The purpose of this chapter was to review various aspects of education for the hearing-impaired child. It is clear that the changes in federal educational provisions for the hearing-impaired child represent a considerable challenge to today's audiologists. The emphasis is now on the early identification and management of hearing impairment, preferably prior to 2 years of age. Nevertheless, we find that hearing loss poses a significant threat to educational achievement. Even the milder forms of hearing loss have been shown to inhibit educational progress. These ever-increasing changes in the field of education for the hearing impaired result in expanding responsibilities for both the speech-language pathologist and the audiologist working in a school setting.

References

1. United States House of Representatives 99th Congress, 2nd Session. Report 99–860. Report Accompanying the Education of the Handicapped Act Amendments of 1986.
2. Davis JM, Elfenbein J, Schum R, Bentler RA: Effects of mild and moderate hearing impairments on language, educational and psychosocial behavior of children. *J Speech Hear Disord* 51:60, 61, 1986.

Suggested Readings

The Commission on Education of the Deaf: *Toward Equality: Education of the Deaf.* (A Report to the Congress of the United States) Washington, DC, U.S. Department of Health, Education, and Welfare, 1988.

Baker C, Cokely D: *American Sign: A Teachers' Resource Text on Grammar and Culture.* Silver Spring, MD, TJ Publishers, 1980

Bess FH, McConnell FE: *Audiology, Education, and the Hearing-Impaired Child.* St. Louis, CV Mosby, 1981.

Bess FH: Unilateral sensorineural hearing loss in children. *Ear Hear* 7 (no. 1, special issue): 1–54, 1986.

Caccamise F, Newell W: A review of current terminology used in deaf education and signing. *Journal of the Academy of Rehabilitative Audiology* 17, 106–129, 1984.

Davis J, Shephard N, Stelmachowicz P, Gorga M: Characteristics of hearing impaired children in the public schools. Part II. Psychoeducational data. *J Speech Hear Disord* 46:130–137, 1981.

Davis JM, Elfenbein J, Schum R, Bentler RA: Effects of mild and moderate hearing impairments on language, educational and psychosocial behavior of children. *J Speech Hear Disord* 51:53–62, 1986.

DiFrancesca S: Academic achievement test results of a national testing program for hearing impaired students. United States: Spring 1971. Series D, no. 9, Annual survey of hearing impaired children and youth. Washington, DC, Office of Demographic Studies, Gallaudet College, 1972.

Feagans L: Otitis media: a model for long term effects with implications for intervention. In Kavanuagh JF (ed): *Otitis Media and Child Development*. Parkton, MD, York Press, 1986.

Moores DF: *Educating the Deaf—Psychology, Principles and Practices*, ed 3. Boston, Houghton Mifflin, 1987.

Oyler RF, Oyler AL, Matkin ND: Unilateral hearing loss: demographics and education impact. *Language, Speech and Hearing Services in Schools* 19:201–209, 1988.

Quigley SP, Thomure FE: Some effects of hearing impairment upon school performance. Springfield, IL, Office of Education, 1968.

Schien JD, Delk MT: The deaf population of the United States. Silver Spring, MD, National Association of the Deaf, 1974.

INDEX

Page numbers in *italics* denote figures; those followed by "t" denote tables.